FRACTURES
IN CHILDREN

FRACTURES
IN CHILDREN

WALTER PUTNAM BLOUNT, A.B., M.D., F.A.C.S.

Clinical Professor of Orthopaedics, Marquette University School of Medicine. Attending Staff Surgeon, Columbia Hospital, Johnston Emergency Hospital, Milwaukee; Consulting Staff, Milwaukee County Hospital; Member of the American Orthopaedic Association, American Academy of Orthopaedic Surgeons, Société Internationale de Chirurgie Orthopédique et de Traumatologie, Honorary Member, Deutsche Orthopädische Gesellschaft.

THE WILLIAMS & WILKINS COMPANY

BALTIMORE   •   1955

COMPOSED AND PRINTED AT THE
WAVERLY PRESS, INC.
BALTIMORE 2, MD., U. S. A.

To my father,

Ralph Earl Blount,

my first and most generous

teacher

Preface

This book is a composite of the experience of the members of the Fracture Service of the Milwaukee Children's Hospital over a period of more than twenty years. Its delayed appearance has worked a tremendous advantage to all concerned. Our mature experience with end results has enabled us to formulate rules and enumerate principles of treatment. The discussions following numerous lectures in various parts of the country have promoted clear thinking and simplified the statement of these principles. The surgeons in attendance at these lectures and the Instructional Courses have submitted invaluable material. I have quoted freely from many published works and have given the references, but have made no attempt to furnish a complete bibliography. My thanks are due to all who have increased the scope of this book, and who have aided in condemning unnecessary and ill-advised operations on children.

Fractures of the skull and craniocerebral injuries are in the domain of the specialist in neurosurgery. Dr. David Cleveland, of Milwaukee, has contributed a thoughtful chapter on this subject which prepares the general physician or the general surgeon to deal with emergencies and treat the simpler head injuries. His splendid contribution will be a ready reference for those who must deal with head injuries in children.

No less specialized is the treatment of face injuries. Dr. William H. Frackelton, of Milwaukee, has covered this subject admirably and in enough detail to make his section an adequate guide for those who treat the simpler injuries. It will aid them in the recognition of the more serious injuries that must be transferred to a specialist for treatment.

Although the treatment of hand injuries should be the province of all orthopaedists, it must be conceded that the orthopaedic and other surgeons who have made a special study of hand surgery have the most to contribute to our knowledge of this subject. I am pleased to include another chapter by Dr. William H. Frackelton, past president of the American Society for Surgery of the Hand, whose originality and sound judgment bring much that is new and yet eminently practical to the treatment of hand injuries in children.

Dr. Irwin Schulz was formerly one of the moving spirits of the Fracture Service at the Milwaukee Children's Hospital. Many of the most astute observations included in this book are the product of his clear thinking. He has done pioneer work in the treatment of wringer injuries and the section on this subject was contributed through his collaboration.

To all of the past and present members of the Orthopaedic Section and the Fracture Services of the Milwaukee Children's Hospital and, in particular, my colleague, Dr. Albert C. Schmidt, and my associate, Dr. Robert H. Cassidy, and the resident staff who have so faithfully followed the cases so that we may have end results to study, I owe my thanks. I am grateful to the Department of Radiology of the Milwaukee Children's Hospital and particularly to the Chairman of the Section, Dr. Hans W. Hefke, whose keen observations and sound advice over the years have contributed much to our understanding of fractures in children. I am no less grateful to Dr. S. A. Morton and the Department of Radiology of Columbia Hospital for the contribution of some of the more unusual cases.

The Williams & Wilkins Company has been most patient. Thanks to them for a technical job well done. To Miss Dorothy Thiel, my most valued nurse and technician goes the credit for most of the better roentgenograms, and to Mr. Carl Brill, my appreciation for the excellent drawings. Miss Mary Dougherty of the Milwaukee Academy of Medicine has worked long on the references. Dr. Paul Arneson's assistance has been invaluable in reading copy and proof.

Miss Marion Kline, who has been my right hand for as long as we have studied fractures in children, really wrote the book—many times. If it is well written, it is due to her effort and your thanks should be added to mine.

To all who have helped I am grateful: the succession of administrators, record librarians, physical therapists, orthopaedic nurses, and technicians. And finally may I express my incalculable debt to my wife, for without her sympathetic understanding and encouragement this book would not have been written.

WALTER P. BLOUNT

Contents

Because the illustrations in this book utilize so much more space than the text, it was impracticable to follow the usual custom of interspersing text with pictures, except in the first chapter. In later chapters the text is first presented, followed by the pictures appertaining to the chapter. In a few cases, where reference is made in the text to a picture *not* immediately following, the page number of the picture so referred to is given, for the convenience of the reader.

CHAPTER I

Introduction

A book about fractures in children is needed by the general physician, the general surgeon, and, I fear, many orthopaedists. Children's fractures are as different from those of adults as are their metabolic and psychic problems. The separate consideration of children's fractures does not complicate the issue, but simplifies it. Differential diagnosis is more important than in adults. Epiphyseal lines, rarefaction produced by blood vessels, dense growth lines, congenital fractures and pseudofractures, unique pathologic fractures, and a host of other phenomena appear on the roentgenograms to confuse the surgeon. I have devoted many pages to the diagnosis and treatment of lesions which look something like fractures in children.

Before-and-after films are adequate to demonstrate the treatment of adult fractures. The growth factor in children alters the picture as time marches on. I have used numerous serial roentgenograms to illustrate these variations and the changes of treatment that are necessary.

Adults are exposed to a great variety of injuries with a correspondingly complicated etiology and fracture pattern. Their bones break increasingly easily with advancing years so that complex fractures are likely. Except for transportation and farm machinery accidents, the causes for bone injuries in children are usually simple. The bone changes are characteristic and the outcome predictable. The principles of treatment are correspondingly simple. The fact that most fractures in children heal fairly well with indifferent treatment has led the unwary to neglect the fact that other fractures terminate disastrously unless expertly handled. Some papers have made valuable contributions to our knowledge but others have been misleading. Monographs by Ashhurst (1) and Truesdell (2) have been important milestones. The subject of children's fractures has been somewhat neglected in recent years because there has been no economic stimulus to make end result studies like the urge to evaluate the compensable accidents of industry.

The diagnosis is complicated in infants by the lack of an accurate history, and by the lack of cooperation during the examination. Even the roentgenogram is difficult to interpret because the ends of the long bones are composed largely of cartilage. The osseous centers appear at predictable ages which have been charted (Figs. 1 and 2). In older children the epiphyseal plates introduce translucent lines which are sometimes difficult to distinguish from fractures. Fractures through the epiphyseal plates are difficult to recognize if there has been a spontaneous reduction. Thurston Holland's (3) sign of a triangular chip of metaphysis attached to the epiphysis on the side to which the epiphysis was previously displaced is reliable when present, particularly at the distal end of the radius (Fig. 139, p. 102).

Most important in this connection and in general when taking roentgenograms of children is the rule: Always take both right and left parts in similar positions and each, of course, in two projections. Compare the roentgenograms of the injured extremity carefully with those of the uninjured. Failures to observe this rule are responsible for most of the errors in diagnosis of children's fractures. A greenstick fracture in a child may show only a wrinkle in the cortex, visible only when projected in profile. The torus fracture of the distal end of the radius is an example (Fig. 106, p. 80).

At certain stages of a child's development minor twists and tumbles will cause fractures of the long bones that do not occur in adults. On the contrary, severe trauma to the torso is required to produce spinal or pelvic fractures which are common in adults with lesser injuries. The appearance of multiple fractures without adequate trauma suggests at once the existence of a deficiency disease like osteogenesis imperfecta. Isolated spontaneous fractures in children are likely due to benign bone cysts (Chapter XVII, Pathologic Fractures).

As compared to the differences of opinion with regard to the treatment of fractures in adults there is relative unanimity among the few men who have studied the problem in children. The principles of treatment are simple (142). Alignment is the chief requirement. The fracture should not be grossly angulated or rotated. Rotational deformities are inexcusable and should be corrected at an early stage of treatment. Slight angulation is frequently compatible with a perfect end result. This means that many impacted fractures in young children can be immobilized without reduction. On the contrary, angulated greenstick fractures near the center of long bones, particularly the forearm bones of older children, must be completely broken through and accurately aligned if permanent disability is to be avoided.

General rules may be formulated for appraising a deformity and establishing a prognosis following the fracture of a growing bone. The *degree of spontaneous correctability* of angular deformities in long bone fractures of children is dependent upon several factors:

(A) *Three local variables:* (I) The age of the child; (II) The distance of the fracture from the end of the bone; (III) The amount of angulation. The younger the child and the nearer to the end of the bone, the more angulation one may accept. The older the child, and the nearer the fracture is to the middle of the bone, the more accurate the reduction must be.

(B) The most complete spontaneous correction of angular deformity occurs when the *angulation is in the plane of motion of a neighboring ginglymus joint.* Just proximal to the hinge joints of the knee, elbow, and fingers, angulation with the apex toward the flexor surface produces surprisingly little immediate disability. There is some limitation of flexion but usually this is not noticed by the patient. Hyperextension is insignificant, if present at all. Function is eventually normal unless the fracture occurs near the end of the growth period. Angulation in other directions is likely to persist, at least in part. Rotational deformities are permanent.

(C) *Deformities of or near the femoral neck* are not corrected by molding. The proximal end of the femur is unique in its component struts and levers. In a growing child the results following a trochanteric or subtrochanteric fracture are complex. Apposition is of little significance since nonunion is unknown. Molding cares for local irregularities of form. True to the preceding rule (A) of acceptability of malunions in children, angular deformity near the proximal end of the shaft of the femur tends to straighten out with longitudinal growth. But the change in the angle of the femoral neck with reference to the shaft persists (Fig. 211, p. 165). If the fracture produces a coxa vara, this deformity is permanent. Except as altered by physiologic derotation, rotational malalignment is also permanent.

Similarly an angulation osteotomy below the trochanter in a child will tend to straighten out with growth but the changed relationships of the neck and the shaft persist. Coxa vara is permanently corrected in a young child by subtrochanteric osteotomy but a similar angulation osteotomy gradually loses its buttressing effect in stabilizing a dislocated hip (4). The effect of rotational osteotomy in the subtrochanteric region is permanent.

Apposition (the amount of end to end contact or engagement of the ends of the fragments) and moderate *shortening* are of little significance in children. Long bones may be allowed to unite with bayonet (side to side) apposition in children as old as ten (female) or twelve (male) years with assurance that molding will produce a normal bone before growth is complete. Side to side apposition produces a rapid strong union. Al-

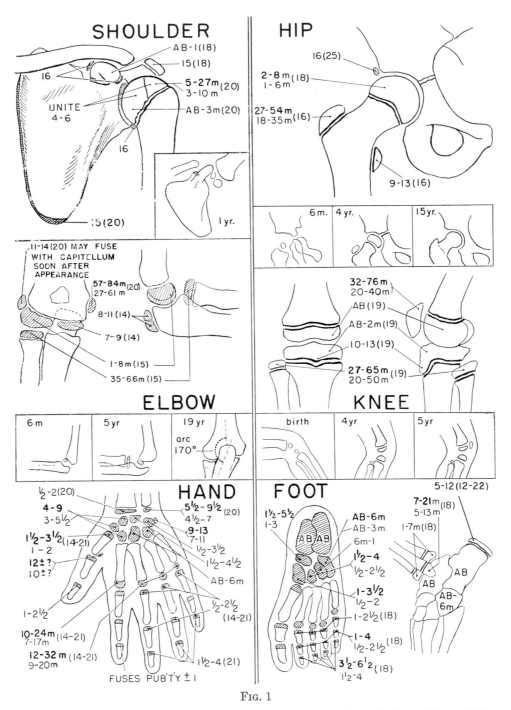

FIG. 1

FIGS. 1 and 2. Range of time of appearance of centers of ossification 10th to 90th percentile. Figures followed by "m" = months; otherwise = years. Where two sets of figures are given for one center, upper heavier number = males, lower lighter number = females. AB = visible at birth. Approximate age of fusion in parentheses. (Reproduced with permission of Dr. B. R. Girdany and The Williams & Wilkins Co.)

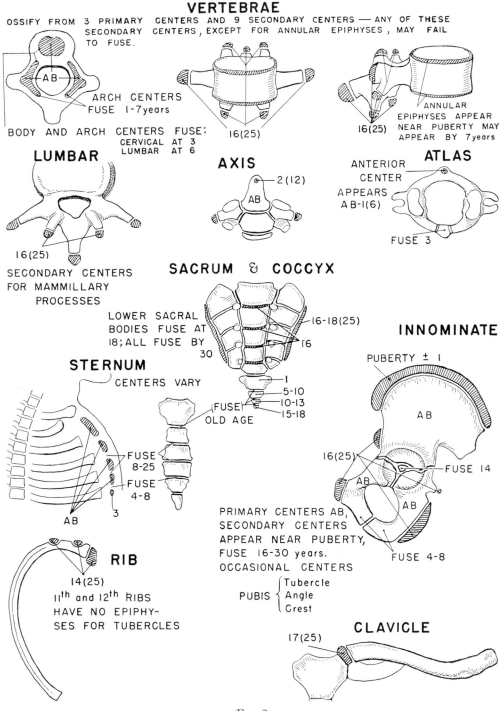

VERTEBRAE

OSSIFY FROM 3 PRIMARY CENTERS AND 9 SECONDARY CENTERS — ANY OF THESE
SECONDARY CENTERS, EXCEPT FOR ANNULAR EPIPHYSES, MAY FAIL
TO FUSE.

ARCH CENTERS
FUSE 1-7years

BODY AND ARCH CENTERS FUSE:
CERVICAL AT 3
LUMBAR AT 6

16(25)

ANNULAR
EPIPHYSES APPEAR
NEAR PUBERTY MAY
APPEAR BY 7years

16(25)

LUMBAR

16(25)

SECONDARY CENTERS
FOR MAMMILLARY
PROCESSES

AXIS

2(12)

AB

ATLAS

ANTERIOR
CENTER
APPEARS
AB-1(6)

FUSE 3

SACRUM & COCCYX

LOWER SACRAL
BODIES FUSE AT
18; ALL FUSE BY
30

16-18(25)

16

1
5-10
10-13
15-18

(FUSE)
OLD AGE

INNOMINATE

PUBERTY ± 1

AB

16(25)

AB

FUSE 14

AB

STERNUM

CENTERS VARY

FUSE
8-25

FUSE
4-8

AB   3

PRIMARY CENTERS AB,
SECONDARY CENTERS
APPEAR NEAR PUBERTY,
FUSE 16-30 years.
OCCASIONAL CENTERS

PUBIS { Tubercle
        Angle
        Crest

FUSE 4-8

RIB

14(25)
11th and 12th RIBS
HAVE NO EPIPHY-
SES FOR TUBERCLES

CLAVICLE

17(25)

FIG. 2

though this position is usually not acceptable in adults, it is not only permissible but desirable in displaced fractures of the femur and humerus
of younger children. The stimulus that follows a fracture results in accelerated longitudinal growth of the bone involved and sometimes of another
distal to it. The result is similar to that observed in bones with chronic
osteomyelitis. The mechanism is not entirely clear and the results are not
accurately predictable but the average overgrowth of the individual bones
following displaced fractures may be used as an index of the desirable
overlap during healing (Chapter VII). The end result will be better if the
overgrowth is corrected in advance, because a bone that is too long is
just as disabling as one that is too short. There is no beneficent force
which brings about a "compensatory" (5) shortening (Chapter VII, Injuries of the Femur).

With the desiderata so simplified, definite *principles of treatment* can be
outlined. In most cases, excellent results are obtained by traction or
closed reduction and a cast. When overlapping is desirable, traction is
the method of choice. Fractures near joints are much more frequently
treated successfully by manipulative reduction and plaster immobilization than in adults.

There are definite and predictable exceptions to the success of conservative treatment. These exceptions include three relatively common
fractures about the elbow and a few rare articular fractures. These will
be enumerated and definite principles of treatment outlined under the
various anatomic headings. Open reductions of other fractures are difficult to justify. For lack of knowledge of sound conservative principles or
to suit the convenience of the surgeon, unnecessary operations may have
been done for years without serious complication. But even one unnecessary tragedy in a lifetime is reason enough to abandon such vicious
operations.

A knowledge of *prognosis* which is valuable in adults is of the utmost
importance in children who are going to continue to grow. It is this
growth factor which makes fractures in children so different from those in
adults. Further growth is usually a help in the correction of the deformities of bones that have united in a crooked position or with shortening.
All too frequently, growth is an inexorable force which produces deformity when the epiphyseal cartilage has been damaged. These favorable and
disastrous changes are predictable and should be understood by anyone
who treats fractures in children.

In general, *epiphyseal fractures* are best treated by closed methods. An
exception is at the proximal end of the femur. This subject is discussed
with reference to fractures of the different bones particularly the distal
end of the tibia and radius. A violent longitudinal thrust producing a

crushing injury to the epiphyseal plate will cause retardation of epiphyseal growth and serious deformity. Unless there has been damage to
the growing cells of the epiphyseal plate at the time of injury, slight overgrowth is the rule, retarded growth an exception. After two weeks, considerable displacement is usually to be preferred to forceful closed reduction or an open reduction.

The questions have often been asked, "How soon will such a deformity
show up? When can we be relatively sure that there has been no serious
injury to the growing cells of the epiphyseal plate?" These questions
cannot be answered in a few words. It is not "how long", but "how much"
growth" that determines the answer. The elongation of bones occurs un-
predictably in spurts. If the fractured one and its fellow on the opposite
side grow little or not at all in a given interval, the answer must be postponed.

My advice would be as follows: When an epiphysis has been injured,
take simultaneous roentgenograms of the affected bone and the one on
the opposite side at six foot distance. The length should be accurately
recorded. If, after three months or six months, the measurements of a
roentgenogram similarly taken, show that there has been appreciable
growth, and that the rate on the fractured side is the same or a little
faster than on the opposite side, then one can safely say that the epiphysis has not been damaged. If there has been no appreciable growth,
then one just doesn't know. If the fractured bone has grown less, then
one should give a guarded prognosis and repeat the roentgenograms at
two month intervals.

It doesn't mean anything to say "After six months", because bones
may rest six months without growing appreciably. It doesn't mean anything to know that "The child has grown one inch in height" because
occasionally the addition to height is entirely in the torso while the extremities grow very little, if any.

The technic of reduction and particularly that of fixation varies somewhat with the age of the child, but differs greatly from the technic in
adults. Nonunion may be ignored as a complication if open operation is
avoided. Fixation is needed for a much shorter time than in adults; the
duration being roughly proportional to the child's age. Immobilization
should be efficient in order to prevent deformity. Children are much more
active than the older members of their families and their broken bones
must be held even more securely. In general, it is wise to immobilize one
or more joints on either side of the fracture until the callus is solid. Permanent stiffness of joints due to such immobilization is unknown in
children. Skin traction may be applied to straight fingers for three weeks
without causing residual stiffness. Persistent limitation of joint motion

near a fracture is due to bony deformity and/or fibrosis of the soft parts resulting from the initial trauma or rough and repeated manipulations. Early mobilization is not only unnecessary but is contraindicated. Let the soft parts heal. Keep the part at rest until the bone fragments are solidly united.

Physical therapy, which is invaluable in the treatment of injured adults, is almost never necessary in the management of uncomplicated children's fractures. Basic principles of physiology and mechanics must be followed by the doctor in charge of the case. Reduction is gentle to avoid soft tissue damage. Casts, splints, bandages, and traction are applied with the part in a comfortable position. There must be no obstruction to circulation. Ice is applied locally and the part elevated to minimize swelling. Heat and massage would be wasted and passive manipulation does more harm than good. At the proper time active motion is supplied by the healthy child in unlimited quantities. Early passive motion which was strongly urged even as late as Ashhurst's day (1) should be strictly taboo.

At the elbow where there is frequently a delay in the return of motion, a "hands off" policy must be followed for many months. If the fracture is properly reduced, solidly healed, and there is no complicating fibrosis of the joint capsule, normal motion will return. The child knows instinctively better than his parents, physical therapist, or doctor what he may do without harm. Pain is his guide to restriction of activity. It is a good one. If left to his own devices, he will recover in the shortest possible time. Any attempt to hasten the return of motion by loading with pails of sand or manipulating, prolongs the restriction of motion indefinitely by perpetuating the protective spasm. In children there is no place for manipulation under anesthesia. If extensive fibrosis prevents the return of motion, an operation is necessary to excise the fibrosed tissue (6). Increased extension may be obtained by a wedged cast or manipulation but usually the gain will be only temporary. The child's attempts at normal function plus "tincture of time" will produce the maximal permanent improvement that can be obtained without the aid of surgery.

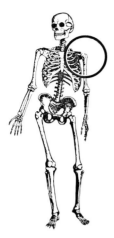

CHAPTER II

Injuries of the Shoulder Girdle

FRACTURES OF THE CLAVICLE

It should be no surprise that the clavicle is one of the most frequently fractured bones in the body, particularly during childhood. It serves as the only bony connection between the shoulder girdle and the trunk. Except for its articulation with the sternum, the shoulder girdle floats in a sea of muscles. Any medially directed blow on the shoulder is transmitted to the clavicle. This bone is likely to be the one to break when the force is applied to the outstretched hand, the elbow, or the shoulder. This means that the clavicle is subject to injury with almost any childhood accident.

Fractures at Birth and During Infancy

Compression of the shoulder girdle during delivery will occasionally cause a fracture of the clavicle (2). If the force is great, the fracture may be displaced with overriding. A mother may roll on a newborn infant causing a similar fracture. Sometimes an infant is dropped on the shoulder, or beaten by a mentally incompetent parent with sufficient force to produce this fracture.

The common symptom is pseudoparalysis of the arm with obvious pain when the arm is moved on the affected side. If the fracture is complete, the pain will be considerable. A newborn infant with a greenstick fracture may be moved more freely. Rest in the supine position is all the treatment necessary.

The symptoms of a displaced fracture may be relieved in the toddler by the addition of a figure of eight bandage of flannelette. Overriding of 5 mm. and angulation of 10° may be accepted. More deformity than this is not encountered. Healing is very rapid and the fracture may be ignored after ten days.

9

Frequently a greenstick fracture is not discovered until massive callus has formed. The explanation of the child's previous fussiness is then evident. The mother should be assured that the bump will disappear entirely in a few months.

In *pseudoparalysis of the arm*, the physician is likely to suspect the humerus rather than the shoulder girdle because the child guards the arm so carefully, and the true diagnosis is revealed for the first time by the roentgenogram.

Reduction is rarely necessary in *a child under six years*, even if the fracture is displaced (Fig. 26, p. 24). Grotesque roentgenographic appearance is characteristic due to the complex curve of the bone, and is compatible with an excellent cosmetic and functional result (Fig. 27, p. 25). In the rare case with gross overriding, temporary lateral traction on the arm with elevation of the bed on the affected side may be desirable (Fig. 12, p. 17). A child of three to six cannot be kept flat in bed. A figure-of-eight bandage of stockinet, partially filled with sheet wadding (Fig. 3) may be tightened every morning by the mother. It will give comfort and is all the support necessary.

Fractures of the Clavicle in the Child Six to Twelve Years Old

As the child grows older, games and sports account for falls on the elbow or shoulder with a direct medial thrust on the end of the clavicle. Greenstick fractures are still frequent but overriding fractures are more common.

The greenstick fracture is well treated by the cotton figure-of-eight dressing (Fig. 3). The infant should wear the support for three weeks, the older child, for four. The markedly displaced and overriding clavicular fracture of the older child should be reduced. Satisfactory anesthesia is obtained by injecting procaine into the hematoma. The child is seated in a chair and tied securely in place. A bolster is placed behind the small of the back. This position is ideal for the reduction (Fig. 4). To maintain the position, soft, all wool felt is fitted as a figure-of-eight and over this plaster slabs and then turns of plaster are added to complete the yoke popularized by Billington (7). While the plaster is still soft, it should be molded to form a rope in either axilla and should be pulled away from the back of the neck. This is the most comfortable of the secure dressings for a fracture of the clavicle in a child (Fig. 6).

The prognosis is uniformly good. The "bump" of callus and the alarming "deformity" frequently seen in the roentgenogram will be obliterated by the molding incident to further growth (Fig. 28, p. 25). There is no justification for open reduction.

Fractures of the Scapula

Direct violence and particularly automobile injuries are responsible for most of the displaced fractures of the scapula. Blows from hard objects and falls on the back of the shoulder will produce lesser fractures.

The treatment is conservative even when there is considerable displacement. Simple rest of the shoulder girdle with a sling and a swath is sufficient. Fracture of the scapula is frequently combined with other injuries necessitating bed rest. In such a case, the fractured scapula may be ignored so long as the patient is comfortable. Irregularities of contour disappear with further growth. If a bony spicule should persist, it may be removed at a later date. It should be noted that the entire blade of the scapula is removed without loss of function in such conditions as scapula alta and deforming exostosis.

Injuries at the Shoulder Joint

Injuries at the shoulder are caused by falls on the outstretched hand or elbow or sudden traction on the arm. Soft tissue injuries at birth vary from sprains to avulsion of the brachial plexus. In children, dislocations are extremely rare as compared to their frequency in adolescents. Fractures fall into definite anatomic types according to age groups.

Injury at birth from vigorous manipulation of the arm may cause an epiphyseal separation and/or a dislocation which reduces spontaneously (2). Fractures below the epiphyseal plate are likely to be through the middle of the shaft. Shoulder injuries are extremely difficult to diagnose because the head of the humerus is still cartilaginous. The dysfunction associated with a bone injury is often misinterpreted as a brachial palsy. Fracture or dislocation should be suspected when there is marked swelling of the shoulder with pseudoparalysis of the arm even with negative roentgenographic findings. One should always repeat the roentgenogram in a week (8). By that time callus will be evident (Figs. 7, 8) if there is a fracture. A dislocation can be detected by careful comparison of the two shoulders in both the anteroposterior and lateral projections.

One of these injuries is frequently combined with brachial birth palsy. The coexistence of a nerve lesion should not blind one to the presence of a bone injury (9). In particular, one should avoid the mistake of abducting the arm on a splint and redislocating a shoulder which had been reduced spontaneously. A splinted Erb's palsy should always be examined roentgenographically to rule out dislocation of the shoulder.

A rare but characteristic lesion is a complete fracture dislocation of the epiphysis at birth with 180° rotation of the head fragment (Fig. 10). This injury is not often recognized until later. If a diagnostic wizard could recognize the lesion but reduction could not be accomplished by manipulation, open operation would be justified to rotate the humeral head. The deformity resulting from this serious injury is well shown in Figure 10. Although unsightly, the shortening of an upper extremity is of little significance. Function can be greatly improved by an osteotomy (Fig. 11).

In all of these shoulder injuries of the newborn, the treatment is easy compared to the difficulty of recognition of the lesion. Relative immobilization and rest of the part is usually all that is necessary. Brief lateral traction is occasionally helpful as in the treatment of similar injuries in the infant (Fig. 12). The crib may be elevated on the side of the fracture for countertraction. A sling is unsatisfactory in an infant. A collar and cuff is better treatment (Fig. 37, p. 36), and it may be combined with a swath.

Rough handling of an infant may cause the simpler injuries described in the preceding paragraphs. The lesions to be differentiated are a true brachial birth palsy and/or a pseudoparalysis from congenital syphilis or scurvy. The latter two can usually be recognized in a roentgenogram. A true nerve lesion should be evident on testing with a pin. It is a common mistake to treat a brachial birth palsy with a splint in the position of abduction 90°, rotation outward 90° when there is an unrecognized complicating fracture or dislocation. This error may cause permanent dislocation or limitation of motion.

Children from two to seven years sustain injuries at the upper end of the humerus while at play. Dislocations and epiphyseal injuries are rare. A *transverse subtubercular fracture* is common and likely to be greenstick in the younger child. In the latter case, angulation of 10°–15° is compatible with a normal end result and the fracture need not be reduced. A collar and cuff is all the treatment necessary.

The *displaced subtubercular fracture* is normally aligned by the application of a hanging cast (Fig. 13). Bayonet apposition with 1 cm. of overriding is ideal position. Ten to twenty degrees of angulation are permissible. Although the initial appearance is shocking (Fig. 14), molding takes care of the roentgenographic picture (Figs. 15, 16). The shortness is outgrown in a few months. Occasionally following severe trauma such as sustained in an automobile accident, bed rest with lateral traction is desirable. In such a case, care should be taken to avoid malrotation. The best plan is to flex the elbow and have the forearm pointing straight upward from the bed in neutral rotation (Fig. 12). In most instances, a hanging cast with the elbow flexed to 80° should be substituted in a few days so that the child may be ambulatory. The cast may be changed for a collar and cuff or a sling in three or four weeks.

The rationale of the *hanging cast* is simple. The long head of the biceps crosses the shoulder joint. The biceps functions in flexion of the elbow and in supination. Immobilization of the elbow helps to place the shoulder at rest. A padded bandage around the neck supports the wrist and lets the cast hang free (Fig. 13), so as to produce an ideal traction effect. The child should sit up in a semireclining position in a chair or bed for the first night or two. After that he may lie flat in bed. A swath about the chest and cast may increase his comfort for the first few days.

In the child of eight to fourteen years subtubercular fractures are less common and *epiphyseal fractures* of the proximal end of the humerus occur during games and sports (Fig. 17). Dislocations are uncommon until adolescence.

The treatment is conservative. It is the greatest fallacy to think that accurate reduction of an epiphyseal fracture at the proximal end of the humerus is important enough to require open operation (10). Nothing could be farther from the truth. If seen promptly, this fracture can be accurately reduced by closed methods. Usually simple traction and the application of a hanging cast is all that is necessary (Fig. 13). Occasionally it will be found difficult to reduce such a fracture unless the arm is placed in a pivotal position (11). Traction with the arm straight overhead and the elbow flexed to 90° will be found effective for reduction (Fig. 18). If the fragments become displaced when the arm is returned to the side, a light plaster spica should be applied holding the arm in the pivotal position (Fig. 19) for four to five weeks (12).

The younger the child with an epiphyseal fracture, the more displacement may be permitted. A ten year old boy with bayonet apposition of an epiphyseal fracture may be treated conservatively with every assurance that the result will be perfect. At twelve years, 50 per cent apposition is satisfactory but there should be less than 10° of angulation. It is easy to obtain this position by the methods mentioned above. Open reduction is likely to damage the epiphyseal plate and cause shortening as well as some permanent stiffness of the shoulder (13). It is mentioned only to be condemned.

One of the commonest shoulder injuries is caused by a solicitous but ignorant nursemaid or parent of the young child. The toddler is helped across the street by holding one hand. When the opposite curb is reached a vigorous jerk pulls the child up to the sidewalk (Fig. 21). If there is not full cooperation from the child, the shoulder may be overstretched causing an acute sprain. The same mechanism operates when the parents try to keep the child from falling by jerking on the arm. The injury may be of considerable severity. The child characteristically refuses to use the arm. The deltoid may seem to be paralyzed (pseudoparalysis), and the condition has been confused with poliomyelitis. *Pulled shoulder* is diagnosed on the history with a negative roentgenogram, pain on attempted motion of the shoulder, but power in the arm below the shoulder. When the force of the jerk is differently transmitted, *pulled elbow* is the result (Chapter IV).

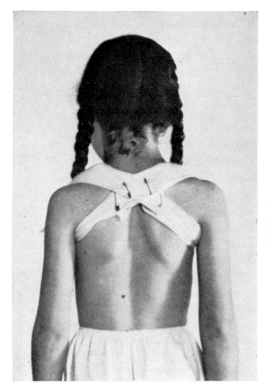

FIG. 3. Fractures of the clavicle without displacement may be treated with a simple figure of eight bandage made of stockinet, padded inside with sheet wadding under the axillae. It is convenient to circle both shoulders and then pin the bandage together in the back rather than to form a figure of eight primarily. The bandage may be tightened each morning by the mother.

FIG. 4. A. A displaced fracture of the clavicle in an older child can well be reduced under local anesthetic with the patient sitting in a chair. A rolled bath blanket is placed at the small of the back. A muslin bandage is passed across the thighs and tied securely to the chair. B. While the shoulders are held upward and back, a strip of felt is formed to a figure of eight and stitched in place. Felt may be enclosed in stockinet if the child is sensitive to wool.

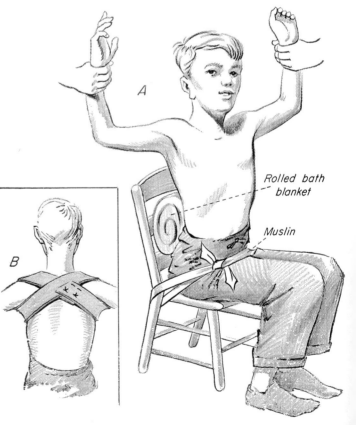

Rolled bath blanket

Muslin

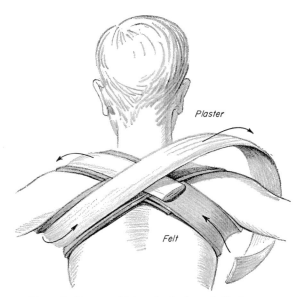

FIG. 5. Long splints of plaster of Paris are secured by turns of plaster bandage. The layers are molded into a rope under the axillae. Firm pressure is made between the shoulder blades so that the weight of the arms is carried here.

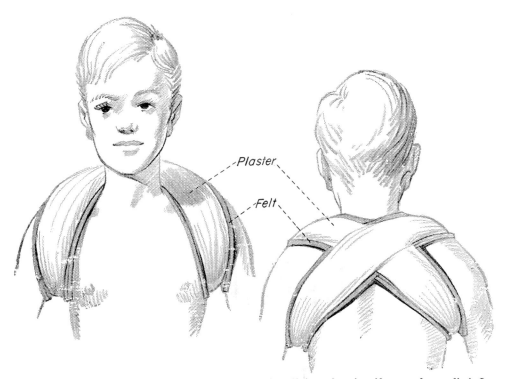

FIG. 6. The completed yoke is a comfortable, efficient dressing if properly applied. It should be worn for four to six weeks.

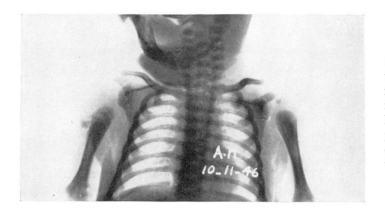

FIG. 7. A. H., male, newborn, 10/11/46. Epiphyseal separation at the proximal end of the right humerus was not recognized until fourteen days after delivery. Callus had begun to form. Note the displacement of the capital osseous center on the right as compared to the left.

FIG. 8. A. H., twelve days after Figure 7. With traction (Fig. 12) satisfactory position was maintained until massive callus formed. Support was no longer necessary.

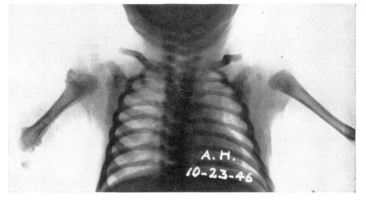

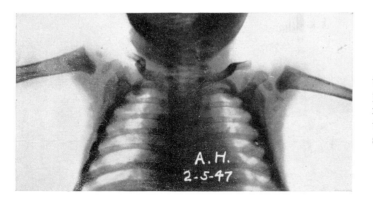

FIG. 9. A. H. Four months after the delivery there is almost complete restoration of the osseous elements of the right shoulder. Note the precocious development on this side.

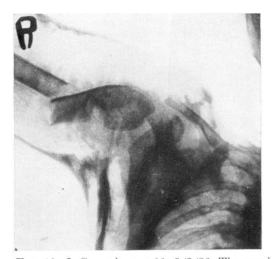

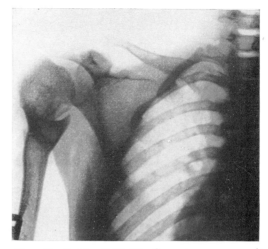

FIG. 10. J. G., male, age 11, 9/2/36. The proximal epiphysis was completely separated at birth. The epiphysis was rotated almost 180° and healed in this position with marked shortening of the arm, limited forward flexion and abduction. This roentgenogram taken at the time of the corrective osteotomy shows the deformity clearly.

FIG. 11. J. G., 6/17/53. Seventeen years after the preceding film shows solid healing and molding of the osteotomy, with greatly improved range in forward flexion and abduction.

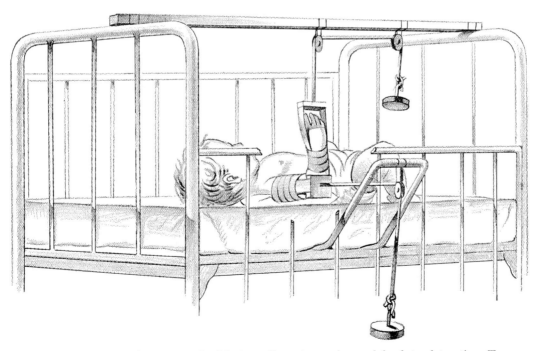

FIG. 12. Flannelette secured with Ace adherent may be used for lateral traction. To prevent rotation of the fragments, the forearm should be suspended perpendicular to the bed.

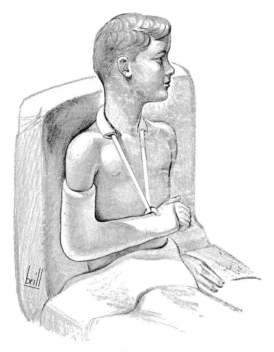

FIG. 13

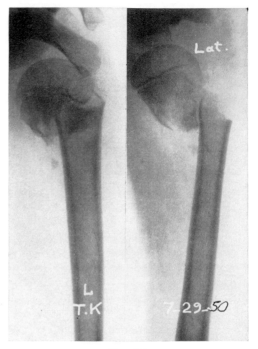

FIG. 14

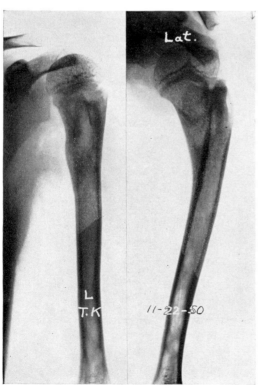

FIG. 15

FIG. 13. A hanging cast may be suspended from the neck with a padded muslin bandage. The elbow should be flexed slightly more acutely than a right angle. The head of the bed must be cranked up for the first few days. [Reproduced with permission of the Journal of the American Medical Association (45)].

FIG. 14. T. K., male, age 7. Epiphyseal fracture of the proximal end of the left humerus. Treatment with a hanging cast and then a sling.

FIG. 15. T. K., four months after the preceding roentgenogram. The child was ambulatory while the fragments healed in bayonet apposition but satisfactory alignment.

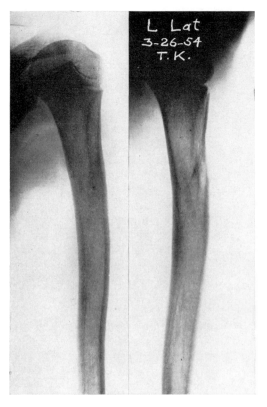

FIG. 16. T. K. Three and one-half years after Figure 15, there is almost complete elimination of the deformity. The humeri were the same length, clinically normal.

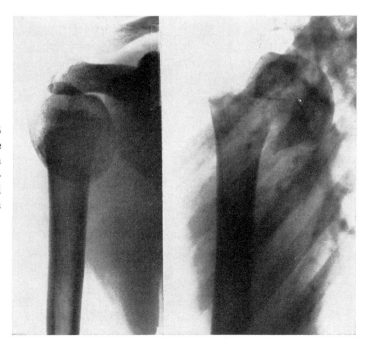

FIG. 17. J. B., male, age 16 4/3/53. Epiphyseal fracture of the proximal end of the humerus with characteristic displacement. The reduction could not be maintained with the arm at the side and open operation was contemplated.

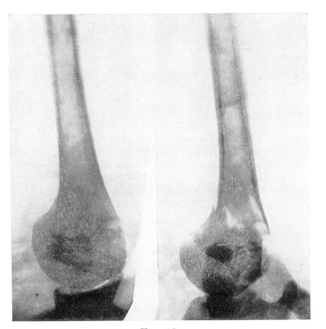

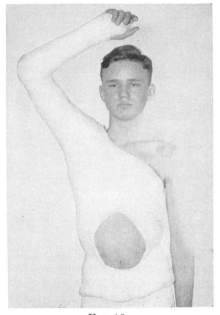

Fig. 18   Fig. 19

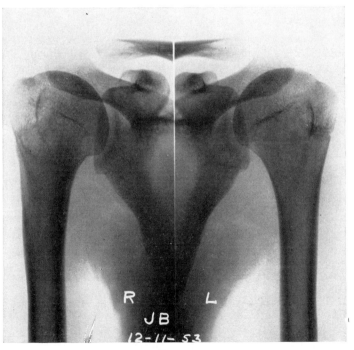

Fig. 18. J. B., 4/6/53, the same fracture as shown in the preceding roentgenograms. Reduction was easily accomplished and maintained by elevating the arm over the head.

Fig. 19. J. B., 4/6/53. A light plaster spica was applied with the arm in the pivotal position. After four weeks the cast was removed and traction applied while the arm was was brought down to the side gradually.

Fig. 20. J. B., 12/11/53. Anteroposterior view of both shoulders eight months after the preceding roentgenogram, showing nearly symmetrical appearance. Function was entirely normal.

Fig. 20

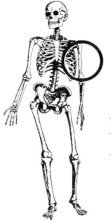

CHAPTER III

Fractures of the Shaft of the Humerus

ETIOLOGY

As compared to the frequency of fractures through the middle of the humerus in adults, this fracture is rather rare in children. It may be a complication of delivery (2). It may occur with rough handling of infants during dressing. In older children it is usually the result of direct trauma. The indirect force of a fall on the outstretched hand or on the elbow causes a fracture elsewhere.

TREATMENT

Fracture of the shaft of the humerus in infancy is ideally treated by lateral traction (Fig. 12, p. 17) for a week. The elbow should be flexed with the forearm pointing straight upward from the bed in neutral rotation to assure the surgeon that a rotary displacement is not occurring. Traction with the forearm straight has allowed rotary displacement particularly in a squirming infant.

When soft callus has formed traction may be discontinued and a collar and cuff with a swath used instead. Apposition is not necessary. Fifteen degrees of angulation are permissible (Figs. 26–28, pp. 24, 25). If there is no displacement, or if traction is not feasible, a collar and cuff with a swath may be used as primary treatment. The infant is less comfortable than with traction.

Ambulatory children are best treated with hanging casts. Two cm. of overriding is not an indication for a change of treatment. One cm. of overgrowth is common in a displaced shaft fracture of the humerus and some overriding is desirable (Fig. 23, p. 23). The rationale of treatment is the same as for fracture of the femur. Bayonet apposition is usually preferable, but a fracture which is not displaced will not overgrow as much and should be left as it is. Healing is very rapid. In four weeks all support

21

may be removed. Reduction is required only in the rare oblique fracture with the bone ends impaled in muscle. Traction under anesthesia is necessary to free the fragments. Traction is then continued or a hanging cast applied. A spica with the arm abducted was common treatment before 1930. It is unnecessarily cumbersome and tends to cause angulation with the apex medially. There is no justification for open reduction.

Complications are almost unheard of in simple fractures of the shaft of the humerus in children. Nonunion is not encountered. Radial nerve palsy which frequently accompanies this injury in adults, occurs very rarely in children. Dr. Cave (14) cited a freak case of radial nerve palsy. A ten year old girl fell in the bathroom catching her arm between the wall and a towel rack. A complete closed transverse fracture of the midshaft of the humerus with minimal displacement was produced by direct trauma. There was immediate loss of power in the radial distribution with hypesthesia to pin prick over the radial sensory area. A cast for six weeks was followed by a cockup splint. Three and one-half months after

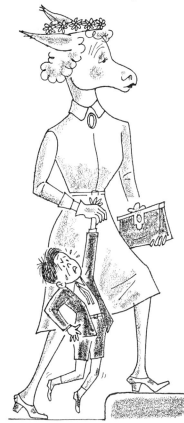

the injury there was electrical but not functional evidence of neurotization. One year following the injury all motions were present except active extension of the thumb. Twenty months after the injury, function was entirely normal.

Fracture of the shaft of the humerus may be one of multiple injuries which confine the patient to bed. Traction is then the best treatment. If the humerus is left in the horizontal position, the elbow should be flexed to insure correct rotation. Occasionally it is better to flex the humerus at the shoulder with skeletal traction through the ulna (Fig. 25, p. 24). Care should be taken that the wire or pin does not damage the epiphyseal plate of the olecranon (15). It is a good plan to apply a cast from the hand to above the elbow to protect the pin from contamination.

Fig. 21. The "jerk" will hurt the child's elbow or shoulder.

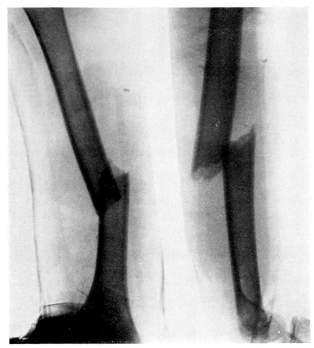

FIG. 22

FIG. 22. W. T., male, age 12, 7/2/36. A fracture of the middle third of the left humerus was complicated by multiple rib fractures and collapse of the left lung. With traction in bed, good alignment was maintained.

FIG. 23. W. T., 9/24/36. Solid union of the fracture with good alignment and 2 cm. overriding three months after Figure 22.

FIG. 24. W. T., 8/23/38, two years after the original injury. The roentgenogram shows persistent changes in the internal architecture but function was entirely normal. There was 1 cm. of shortening.

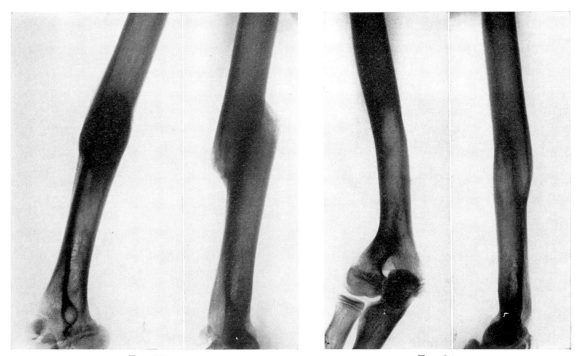

FIG. 23　　　　　　　　　FIG. 24

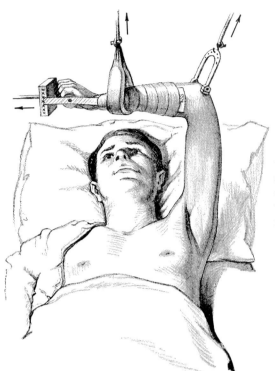

FIG. 25. Traction on the humerus by a Kirschner wire through the olecranon is sometimes used to advantage. Care must be taken to place the wire distal to the epiphyseal plate of the olecranon. If the skeletal traction is to be used for more than a few days, the traction bow should be incorporated in a light plaster cast.

FIG. 26. H. W., male, age 3, 9/19/51. Markedly displaced fractures of the left clavicle and the proximal third of the left humerus caused by the impact of an automobile. The child was first seen six days after the injury. A hanging cast was applied and the deformities permitted to remain.

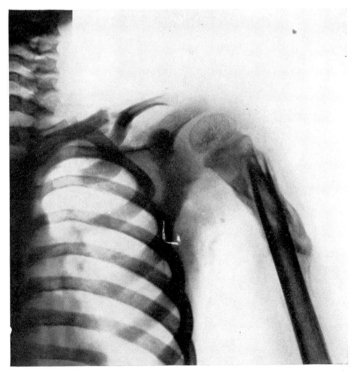

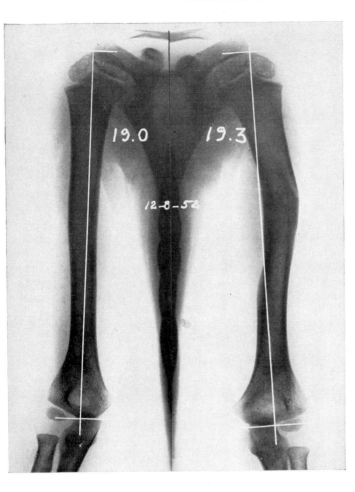

FIG. 27. H. W., 12/8/52, fifteen months following the preceding roentgenogram. The angular deformity and shortening have both been reduced.

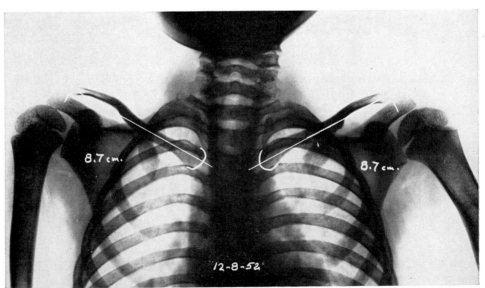

FIG. 28. H. W., 12/8/52. Symmetrical shoulder joints as well as clavicles without deformity in spite of the gross displacement in Figure 26.

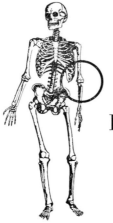

CHAPTER IV

Injuries About the Elbow

SUPRACONDYLAR (DIACONDYLAR, TRANSCONDYLAR) FRACTURES
(60 per cent of elbow fractures)[1]

Etiology

Attempts were made to subdivide these fractures according to the level, in the days when "skiagraphs" were indistinct shadows (65). The more distal ones were called dia-(through) condylar (Fig. 29) or transcondylar and the term "supracondylar" was reserved for those slightly more proximal. But in the lateral view, most fractures look "supracondylar" while in the anteroposterior view, the same fractures have the "transcondylar" appearance. The level through which the break commonly occurs does not vary more than a millimeter or two. The difference, if any, is so slight, that they are grouped together in this book. The exact levels of the fractures do not depend on the age. They occur from three to ten years, with greatest frequency between five and eight. Epiphyseal separation of the entire distal end of the humerus was a common diagnosis at the turn of the century (1). It, too, has vanished with improved radiologic technic.

The supracondylar fracture is characteristically produced by a fall on the outstretched arm with the elbow in hyperextension. If the fracture is complete, the distal fragment is displaced posteriorly, usually with some upward riding (Fig. 30). The deformity may be tremendous so as to simulate a dislocation with which it is commonly confused. If the fracture is incomplete, there is little deformity. Angulation with the apex anteriorly may be sufficient to reduce flexion by 25° to 30° and justify reduction.

Less than 1 per cent of supracondylar fractures are the reverse, or *flexion type*. This injury is produced by a fall on the flexed elbow with

[1] The percentages in this chapter are from end result studies at the Milwaukee Children's Hospital.

26

resultant anterior displacement of the distal fragment (Fig. 33). This flexion fracture should be recognized in order to reduce and immobilize it in sufficient extension to prevent a recurrence of the angular deformity (Fig. 34). It is an error to confuse the types and to treat in extension the usual posteriorly displaced distal fragment, with angulation, apex anteriorly. This mistake causes prolonged hyperextension and limited flexion.

Treatment

If a supracondylar fracture is seen promptly, before swelling has appeared, even though the displacement is extreme, an excellent result is obtained by immediate closed reduction and immobilization in flexion (Fig. 35). If reduction is delayed until there is marked swelling, it is better to apply traction (Fig. 36) in slight flexion rather than to attempt a manipulative reduction. The manipulative method may succeed temporarily even with swelling, but there is little but tradition to recommend it (16). It is seldom possible to flex the elbow sufficiently to maintain reduction without obstructing the circulation, and the position is promptly lost (17). The application of a circular cast is an invitation to Volkmann's ischemia. With three or four days of elevation, traction, and ice packs, the swelling will subside and a manual reduction may be completed under anesthesia.

The introduction of hyaluronidase into fracture treatment has somewhat changed the prognosis in supracondylar fractures. Three to five hundred T.R. units may be injected into the hematoma of a badly swollen elbow. The accelerated dispersion of extra cellular fluid certainly hastens the restoration of the tissues to normal and probably reduces the ultimate fibrous reaction. Theoretically the likelihood of Volkmann's ischemia is reduced. The use of hyaluronidase may make it possible to reduce and maintain the position of supracondylar fractures primarily, even when considerable swelling is present.

Not infrequently, satisfactory position is obtained by Dunlop traction without manipulation. It is particularly indicated in the unstable transcondylar fractures (18, 19). (Fig. 29). One may continue the traction for three weeks and then place the arm in a sling There is usually no need to maintain the traction so long. After ten days when the fracture is reduced and the threat of vascular embarrassment has subsided, I prefer to make the little patient ambulatory by acutely flexing the elbow. This may be done conveniently with rectal pentothal. A collar and cuff maintain the position (Fig. 37).

The ability to reduce but not to hold the position of a supracondylar fracture has influenced some men to use internal fixation. While the results are sometimes good, permanent limitation of motion is all too frequent. This method cannot be justified. With ten days of traction as above, there is enough callus formed to make the fracture "sticky". It will then stay reduced in the flexed position. If there is ever an indication for open reduction in the absence of compounding, it is extremely rare in a fresh case. A considerably greater exposure is necessary than for the open reduction of a lateral condyle. Operations on supracondylar fractures are frequently followed by restricted motion. Blind pinning with protruding pins is always undesirable in children, whose urge to wiggle and scratch cannot be controlled. The use of internal fixation because conservative management fails on the first try is the way of an impetuous surgeon. Patience and gentleness pay off in the treatment of fractures in children, and in supracondylar fractures in particular.

Before the reduction of any elbow fracture, careful examination should establish the normal function of the motor nerves controlling the hand, and the condition of the radial pulse. If the pulse is present, it should not be obliterated by the manipulative reduction. If absent before manipulation, it may be disregarded if the capillary circulation remains good. An absent radial pulse is a danger signal which cannot be ignored, but it is not of itself an indication for open reduction.

The mechanics of closed reduction are simple (Fig. 35). While countertraction is made in the axilla (not by grasping the skin of the arm!) straight traction is made on the supinated hand with one of the operator's hands. The other hand grips the arm just above the elbow with the fingers over the biceps. The thumb lies against the distal end of the proximal fragment while hyperextension is made to disengage the fragments. Malrotation of the fragment is corrected by varying the degree of supination. Lateral displacement is corrected by molding the fragments *before* correcting the posterior displacement. Then the thumb slips down over the tip of the olecranon forcing the hyperextended distal fragment forward into position. Counterpressure is supplied by the fingers. The elbow is flexed to maintain the reduction only after complete reduction of the fracture. The position is checked at once by roentgenograms. If it is not satisfactory, a second reduction may be tried. Traction in bed is preferable to the insult of several manipulations.

Fixation in flexion may be variously achieved (27). The simplest and surest method is to join a collar and cuff by an inelastic bandage (Fig. 37). A light compression dressing about the elbow retards swelling and increases the child's comfort. The addition of a plaster splint to hold the forearm in supination is advocated by some. The rotation of the forearm is actually unimportant once reduction has been obtained and the elbow flexed. Adhesive plaster dressings are secure, too secure. Unless applied with extreme care, they are a threat to the circulation. The worst cases of Volkmann's ischemia have occurred with the use of adhesive plaster or circular casts (Fig. 38).

Following reduction of the supracondylar fracture, the child should be hospitalized for twenty-four hours to insure frequent observation of the circulation of the hand by a competent nurse or house officer. If this is not possible, the parents must understand the danger signals.

Most significant as warnings of early ischemia are: pain, swelling, coldness, cyanosis or pallor, and loss of ability to move the fingers. Remember the triad: Pain, pallor, and paralysis (Fig. 39). The most important and constant of these signs is pain. A well reduced fracture in a child should require no sedation other than aspirin. Pain severe enough to require opiates should be a warning that there is some complication, often too tight a bandage or too much flexion.

Volkmann's Ischemic Contracture

If there is evidence of circulatory embarrassment, the acuity of the flexion is reduced immediately by 20° or 25°. If this change is not instantly successful and there is still a threat of ischemia, all bandages are removed from the elbow and forearm, angulation is reduced to 20°–30° straighter than a right angle, and ice bags applied. Satisfactory position of the fragments and elevation of the forearm are maintained by traction. Usually this is applied to the skin of the forearm without constriction by the use of flannelette strips secured by Ace adherent, (Fig. 36) and held in place by a loosely applied elastic cotton bandage. A Kirschner wire through the olecranon (Fig. 25) (21) is preferred by some. If there are already blebs about the elbow the wire may be inserted in the basal phalanx of the thumb. Loss of position of the fragments is insignificant compared to the tragic disability following unrelieved ischemia (Fig. 38). Prompt blocking of the appropriate sympathetic ganglia is sometimes helpful.

If the symptoms are well advanced or do not subside with conservative measures, no time should be lost before exploring the cubital fossa and volar aspect of the forearm. The tough fascia enclosing the flexor muscles of the forearm is slit permitting the explosive extrusion of edematous muscles and hematoma (22). An injured or markedly constricted brachial artery should be resected. This relieves vasospasm of the collateral arterioles and the reflex involvement of the intimate vasculature of the muscles (23). Delay is disastrous. Within three or four hours, irreversible changes have taken place. The all-too-frequent claw hand usually means inadequate or delayed therapy.

Retention

In the average case, the reduced supracondylar fracture should be immobilized in flexion for three weeks. At the end of that time, the callus is strong enough to allow the elbow to be lowered to a right angle in a sling. In another week or two, all fixation may be discontinued and the child allowed to use the hand at his own discretion (24). It has been adequately proved that more rapid return of normal function will occur if the child is unmolested. Carrying a pail of sand does more harm than good (Fig. 40). There should be no manipulation to increase motion either with or without anesthesia. Repeated stretching of contractures not only distresses the child but perpetuates the spasm and delays the return of normal function.

Occasionally there is an indication to continue traction long enough for union to occur (Fig. 43A). Usually the position will be satisfactory. If there is undesirable angular deformity at the end of three or four weeks, the fracture may still be manipulated under anesthesia and satisfactory position obtained. Bayonet apposition with normal alignment is satisfactory and is not an indication for manipulation at this stage (Fig. 43B). Sharp spicules disappear and contours improve with molding as in fractures near the ends of other long bones (Fig. 44) (25). Angular deformity corrects very little at the distal end of the humerus.

Prognosis

The prognosis in supracondylar fractures must be guarded. If the trauma is not unusually severe, and if the reduction is promptly and gently performed, the result should be a normal elbow (1). There are several chances for disability. The most significant complication, Volkmann's ischemic contracture has been discussed. Exuberant callus will usually disappear spontaneously if unmolested. Physical therapy is not only superfluous but it actually delays recovery (Fig. 45). Myositis ossificans (Fig. 46) occurs most frequently following excessive periosteal stripping, particularly after dislocations. It will usually disappear if unmolested (Fig. 47). Operative removal of the excess bone in children is invariably followed by recurrence. Persistent capsular contracture may require excision of the anterior capsule (6). If osteotomy is necessary to correct extreme angular deformity or to improve the arc of motion it should be postponed for several years.

Reversal of the carrying angle (gunstock deformity) (Fig. 48) may be due to uncorrected medial displacement of the distal fragment (Fig. 49), usually the result of rotation (27). It may follow a perfect reduction and be due to accelerated growth of the lateral condyle; rarely, retarded growth of the medial.

Paralysis from nerve injury is usually only temporary. The radial nerve and occasionally the median may be involved in the absence of ischemia. Early exploration is contraindicated as spontaneous recovery is the rule.

Grossly malunited supracondylar fractures may require open reduction after six to eight weeks (Fig. 50). Moderate permanent limitation of motion is the rule even if reasonably good position can be maintained by pin fixation (Figs. 51, 52). After eight to ten weeks it is usually better judgment to allow the fracture to go untreated and correct the deformity by osteotomy a year or more after the injury.

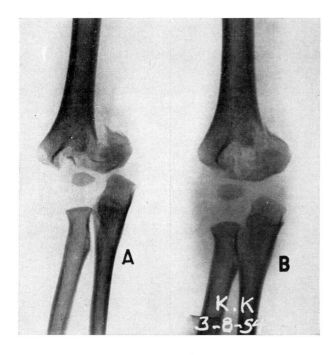

Fig. 29. K. K., male, age 3, 3/8/54. A. A true transcondylar fracture of the distal end of the humerus with displacement of the distal fragment to the ulnar side. B. The reduction obtained by traction as illustrated in Figure 36. The lateral view was also good. After fifteen days a collar and cuff were applied. The boy was discharged from the hospital two days later. At no time was the circulation in jeopardy. Function normal.

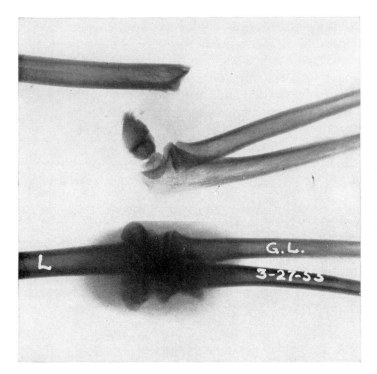

FIG. 30. G. L., male, age 9, 3/28/53. Supracondylar fracture with marked posterior and proximal displacement of the distal fragment, imitating a dislocation on clinical examination.

FIG. 31. G. L., 3/29/53. Antero-posterior and lateral views of the same fracture seen in the preceding figures on the day following an easy reduction. Note the oblique fracture line which makes the fracture trans-condylar in the anteroposterior view but definitely supracondylar in the lateral view.

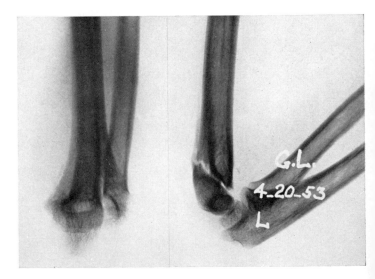

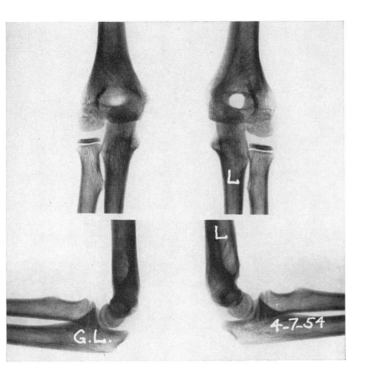

Fig. 32. G. L., 4/7/54, the same case one year after the fracture. Healing has been complete. The internal architecture is restored. The left humerus is 2 mm. longer than the right. Motions and carrying angle are symmetrical.

Fig. 33. C. M., female. Flexion type of supracondylar fracture caused by a fall on the tip of the elbow, four weeks after the arm was immobilized in flexion. Some extension would have improved the position. The end result was a normal elbow.

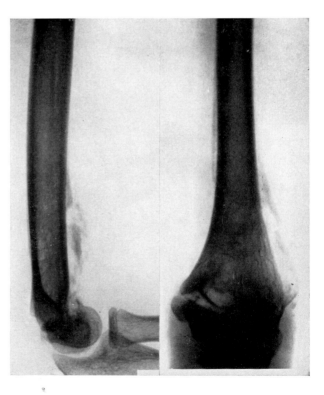

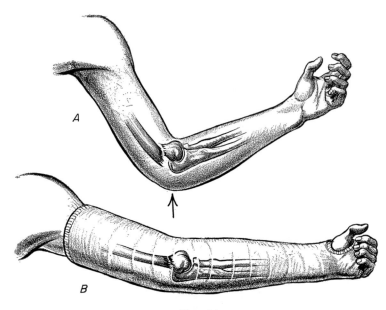

Fig. 34

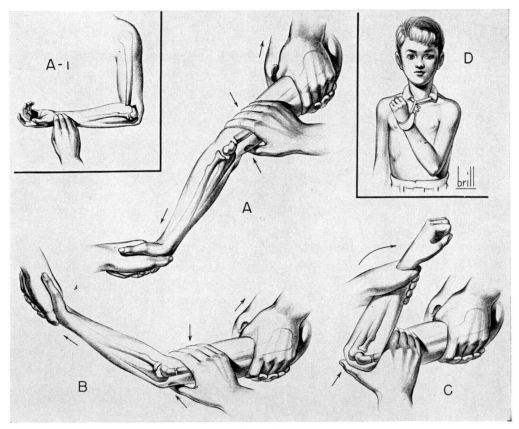

Fig. 35

Fig. 34. A. The mechanism of supracondylar fracture, flexion type. B. Immobilization in some degree of extension is desirable to bring the distal fragment into alignment with the proximal. Immobilization is necessary for only three or four weeks.

Fig. 35. Reduction of a supracondylar fracture. A-. Determine the presence or absence of the radial pulse; examine for motor paralysis. A. Under general anesthesia, apply traction with the elbow hyperextended. Countertraction in the axilla; assistant's hands loosely on the arm. B. The surgeon's thumb forces the distal fragment into position. Accurate reduction is obtained by rotating the forearm and molding the fracture. C. Only after the fracture is completely reduced is the elbow flexed acutely (not forcibly). D. Reduction is maintained by the flexed position, with an efficient collar and cuff. [Reproduced with permission of the Journal of the American Medical Association (45).]

Fig. 36. Dunlop's traction as modified by Allen and Gramse (19) is used temporarily if there is excessive swelling or threatened vascular embarrassment. It may be continued until healing is complete. [Reproduced with permission of the Journal of the American Medical Association (45).]

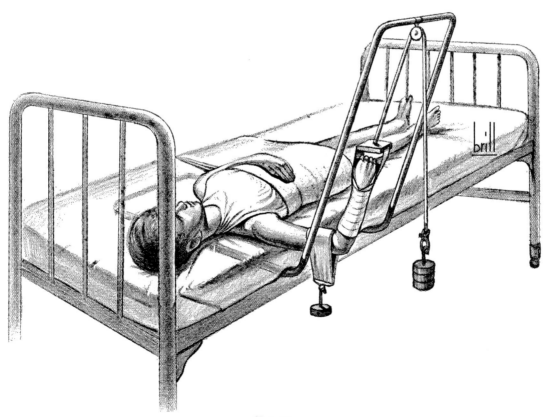

Fig. 36

Fig. 37. A cuff of soft material like wool felt is placed about the wrist and secured with several turns of adhesive plaster. A similar reinforced soft collar is placed about the neck. These are joined by an inelastic bandage with the elbow in acute flexion. It is well to apply a compression dressing to the elbow for a few days. If the child is restless a swath may be added. A plaster slab may be used to maintain supination of the forearm. This is usually superfluous if the fracture has been accurately reduced and the elbow kept flexed.

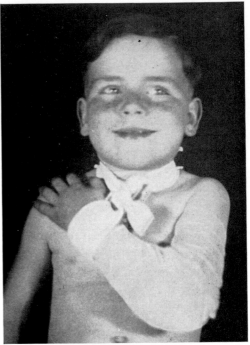

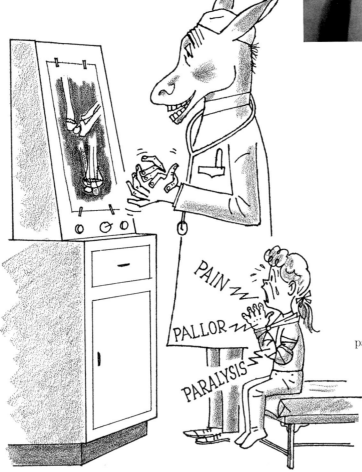

Fig. 39. Doctor, treat the patient, not the picture.

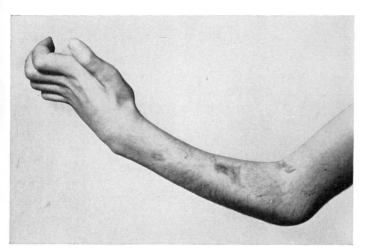

Fig. 38. Volkmann's ischemic contracture. When this stage is reached there has been catastrophic damage to the elbow, forearm, and hand. The warnings were pain, pallor, and paralysis. Prolonged rehabilitation will produce only a very poor substitute for a normal hand and arm.

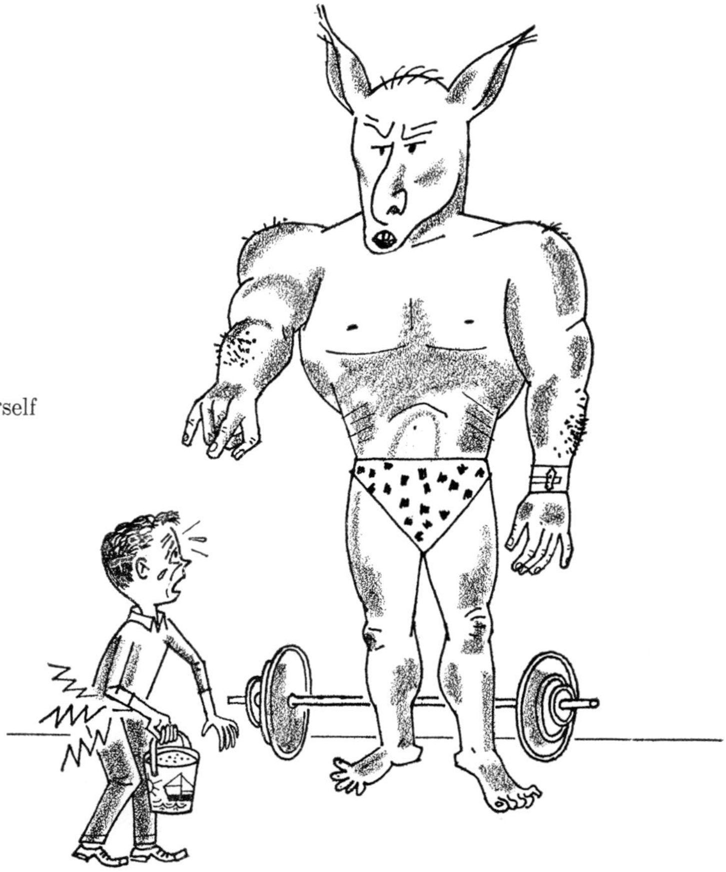

Fig. 40. Carry the sand yourself and let the child get well.

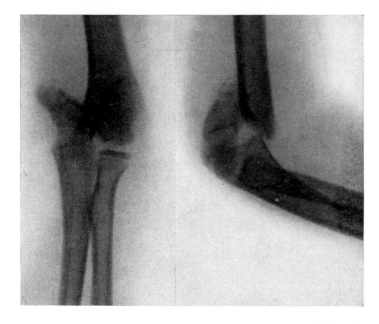

FIG. 41. W. H., male, age 10, 10/27/34. Supracondylar fracture of the left humerus with marked displacement, considerable soft tissue injury, and swelling. [Reproduced with permission of the American Academy of Orthopaedic Surgeons, Instructional Course Lectures (142).]

FIG. 42. W. H., 10/27/34. Accurate manipulative reduction of the preceding fracture. The circulation to the hand was impaired and flexion was released. Dunlop traction was applied. [Reproduced with permission of the American Academy of Orthopaedic Surgeons, Instructional Course Lectures (142).]

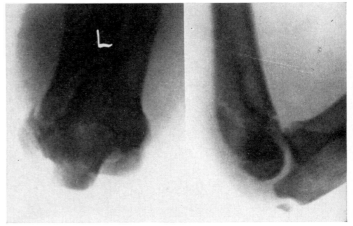

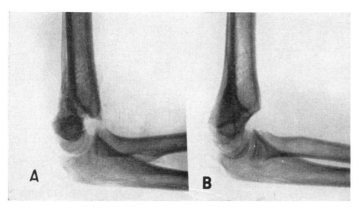

FIG. 43. A. W. H., 11/23/34, the appearance of the preceding fracture after four weeks of traction. There was normal alignment in both views. Apposition was normal in the anteroposterior view; bayonet apposition in the lateral view. B. Seven months later. The spike of bone had absorbed and there was only 10° limitation of flexion. Other elbow motions were normal. [Reproduced with permission of the American Academy of Orthopaedic Surgeons, Instructional Course Lectures (142).]

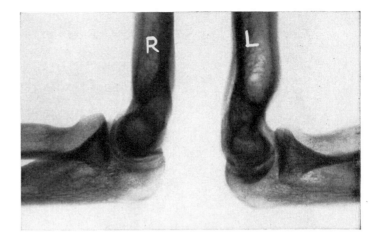

Fig. 44. W. H., 10/3/49, lateral views of both elbows fifteen years later. Slight deformity persists. Except for 10° limitation of flexion on the left, function is normal and symmetrical. No subjective symptoms. [Reproduced with permission of the American Academy of Orthopaedic Surgeons, Instructional Course Lectures (142).]

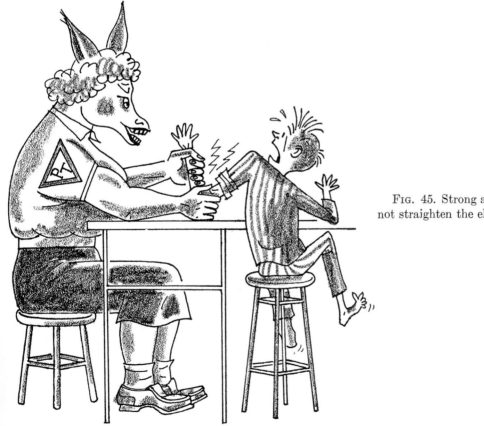

Fig. 45. Strong arm methods will not straighten the elbow.

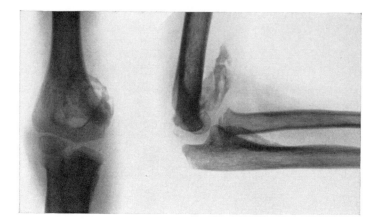

Fig. 46. R. T., male, age 6, 7/19/40. Myositis ossificans following dislocation of the elbow. Motion was greatly restricted. [Reproduced with permission of the Journal of the American Medical Association (45).]

Fig. 47. R. T., 7/17/43, A roentgenogram three years after the preceding. The abnormal bone has almost disappeared. Elbow motions are normal. The treatment was masterly neglect. [Reproduced with permission of the Journal of the American Medical Association (45).

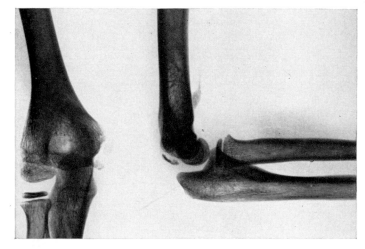

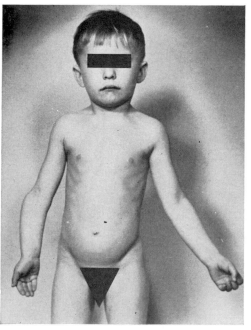

Fig. 48. R. H., male, age 4½, 12/14/42. Gunstock deformity of the right elbow following a supracondylar fracture five months previously. Angulation was due to medial displacement and rotation of the distal fragment.

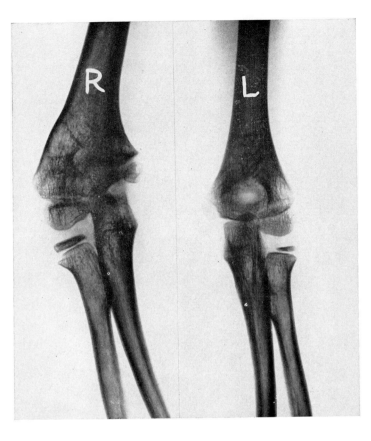

Fig, 49. R. H., 8/26/44. An anteroposterior roentgenogram of both elbows two years after the preceding photograph. There has been no change in the deformity. Note the precocious epiphyseal development on the right. Sometimes cubitus varus is caused by overgrowth of the lateral epiphyseal plate, sometimes by injury of the medial. Lateral and medial angular deformities do not correct spontaneously.

Fig. 50. J. H., male, age 5, 10/17/50. Two views of a grossly displaced and angulated supracondylar fracture of the left humerus six weeks after the injury. Marked deformity, and limitation of flexion 70°, external rotation 30°. Open reduction and pin fixation secured normal position of the fragments.

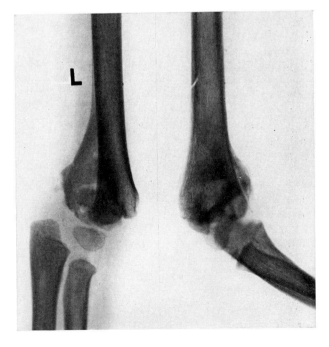

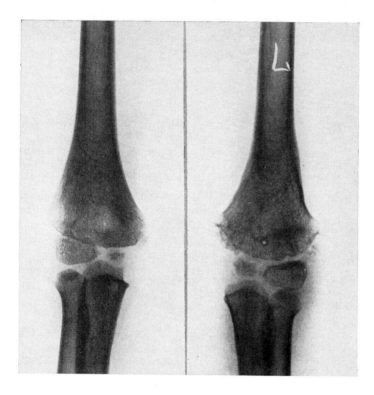

Fig. 51. J. H., 11/7/52, two years after the preceding roentgenogram. There is still 10° limitation of flexion and 25°, of extension.

Fig. 52. J. H., 11/7/52. Normal alignment of the elbows in Figure 51, lateral view. Roentgenograms taken eighteen months later showed improved appearance. Little change on clinical examination. The left humerus is 15 mm. overgrown as the result of the fracture and operation. It is more mature and its epiphyseal plates will close earlier, equalizing some of the overgrowth.

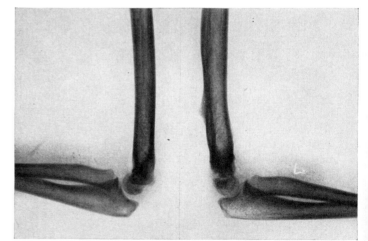

FRACTURES OF THE LATERAL CONDYLE OF THE HUMERUS
(*18.5 per cent of elbow fractures*)

Lateral condylar fractures are produced by hyperextension plus angulation with the apex medially, often a combination of direct and indirect trauma (Fig. 53). The fracture line extends from the lateral epicondyle obliquely downward and medially into the trochlea (Fig. 54A). The deformity is not great and the injury is often dismissed as a sprain, particularly in the infant whose capitellar osseous center has not yet appeared (Fig. 56). Careful palpation of both elbows may be the only diagnostic procedure of any value. When a condylar fracture occurs in combination with a dislocation, there is likely to be prolonged or permanent limitation of motion.

Roentgenograms of both elbows should be taken with symmetrical positioning. Even then the diagnosis is difficult in young children because a large portion of the distal end of the humerus is still cartilaginous. The small oval osseous center of the capitellum may be the only bone visualized in the condylar fragment but usually a flake of metaphyseal bone is carried with it. The fragment is much larger than would appear in the roentgenograms. Its cephalad corner is characteristically rotated laterally and downward in the sagittal as well as the frontal plane, through an arc of 90° or more by the pull of the extensor muscles of the forearm. The fragment is trapped in the joint so that the articular cartilage of the capitellum comes to lie against the raw surface of the metaphysis (Fig. 57). In this position union does not occur.

In some cases with only slight initial displacement, there may be sufficient continuity of the soft parts to hold the fragment in position. Then open reduction is not necessary. The position may be improved by lateral compression of the fragment. Additional roentgenograms should be taken in two days and again at a week because delayed displacement frequently occurs. When the fracture is seen within a few hours of the injury (Fig. 58), a perfect reduction may be obtained by manipulation, particularly if the fragment is large (Fig. 59). If this is accomplished, the elbow should be put up in acute flexion like a supracondylar fracture. Rarely will the position be maintained after the patient wakes up. The fragment is likely to be displaced by the pull of the extensor muscles of the forearm. Its position must be accurately checked by roentgenograms in two planes on the second, fourth and ninth days. If the position is satisfactorily maintained, one may consider himself fortunate (Fig. 60).

If there has been any delay in the reduction or if closed reduction has failed, the patient should be transferred promptly to an institution where an open reduction may be performed satisfactorily. If ideal conditions exist, it is usually wise to operate primarily on the markedly displaced

fracture rather than to subject the patient to the trauma of closed reduction which is likely to fail, or be followed by tardy slipping of the
fragments. Delayed open reductions after the failure of conservative
treatment are less satisfactory (Fig. 61). The operation is more difficult,
limitation of motion persists longer, and loss of the carrying angle from
irritation and overgrowth of the lateral condylar epiphyseal plate is
likely (Fig. 62). Significant arrest or retardation of growth following open
reduction has not been encountered. The limitation of motion which frequently follows an (unnecessary) open reduction of a supracondylar fracture, does not occur after such an operation on a lateral condyle which
requires almost no stripping of soft parts.

The Operation

The open reduction of a lateral condylar fracture is best accomplished
through a Kocher incision (Fig. 57). A tourniquet is not necessary. After
the clotted blood and bone spicules have been removed from the raw surfaces with a curet, the mobile fragment may be rotated and pulled into
position with sharp hooks. An accurate fit should be obtained. Two
ebliquely placed short pins are efficient in holding the fragment. The
periosteum is sutured, but suture alone is rarely enough fixation to prevent some displacement. The pins may be left slightly long so that they
protrude under the skin. After closure of the wound, a cast is applied
from the knuckles to the axilla with the elbow in flexion of 90° and the
forearm in neutral rotation.

At the end of three weeks, the stitches are removed through a window
in the cast. If they have not already pushed through the skin, the pins are
exposed with a pointed knife and pulled out. A week later, the cast may
be removed and replaced by a sling.

Prognosis

Long term (ten to fifteen years) followup of cases treated by prompt
open reduction has shown the results to be uniformly satisfactory. Growth
arrest or significant limitation of motion has not been observed. Delay
makes the operation more difficult. An open operation as late as four
months after the injury should be successful, but moderate deformity is
the rule (Figs. 65–67). Nonunion is not incompatible with satisfactory
function (Figs. 68, 69). If the fracture is older than three months it is
probably wise to allow it to go untreated (Fig. 56) until the patient is full
grown.

If the fracture is unreduced, nonunion invariably occurs (Fig. 71).
There is usually limitation of extension. With longitudinal growth on only
the medial side of the humerus, the carrying angle becomes exaggerated

(Fig. 70). The end result is a painful, weak, deformed elbow. The most significant disability is the delayed ulnar nerve palsy which appears fifteen or twenty years after the injury (Fig. 72).

The deformity is best corrected as soon as growth is complete by osteotomy and excision of the loose fragment (Fig. 73). Pin fixation of the osteotomy is desirable. This operation will relieve the pain of the nonunion and correct the deformity (Fig. 74). Late ulnar nerve symptoms are prevented. If the symptoms are already present, the ulnar nerve may be transplanted to the front of the elbow at the time of the osteotomy. If ulnar palsy is the predominant disability, anterior transposition of the nerve should be done without the osteotomy (28).

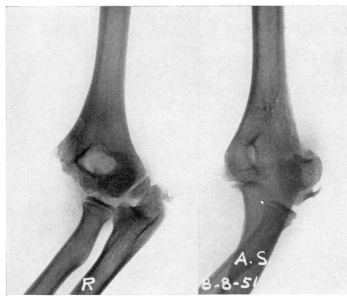

FIG. 53. A. S., male, age 11, 8/8/51. Fracture of the lateral condyle combined with dislocation of the ulnohumeral joint, when he fell off a porch railing landing on his outstretched hand. Ashhurst (1) called this fracture "Posadas" type because it was first described by the professor of surgery by that name at Buenos Aires (26). But this was in the days when "skiograms" were vague shadows. The dislocation was recognized, but the fragment was thought to comprise the entire distal end of the humerus.

FIG. 54. A. S. A. Closed reduction was obtained two hours after the injury under general anesthesia. 8/10/51. A roentgenogram two days after reduction showed accurate maintenance of position. The fracture line was between the arrows. A hanging cast was applied with the elbow in 90° of flexion. B. 10/24/51, ten weeks after reduction. Solid union of the lateral condyle with good position in both views. 70° limitation of extension, 10° limitation of flexion on the right.

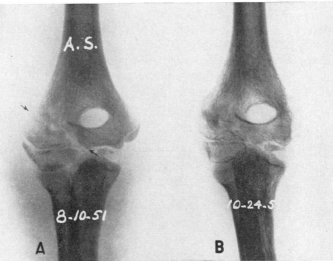

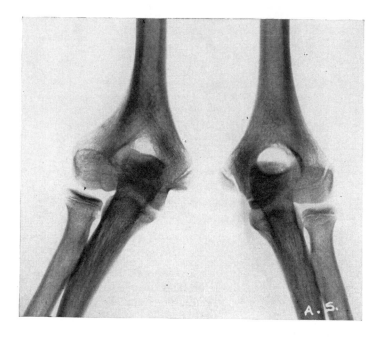

FIG. 55. A. S., 1/13/54, two years after the preceding roentgenogram. Premature closure of the lateral epiphyseal plate had caused 5° increase in the carrying angle. The angle of greatest extension on the right was 180° and on the left was 190°. Other motions were normal; usually they are not. The result was better than that obtained by Ashhurst (1) in his case 28. The injury was apparently identical.

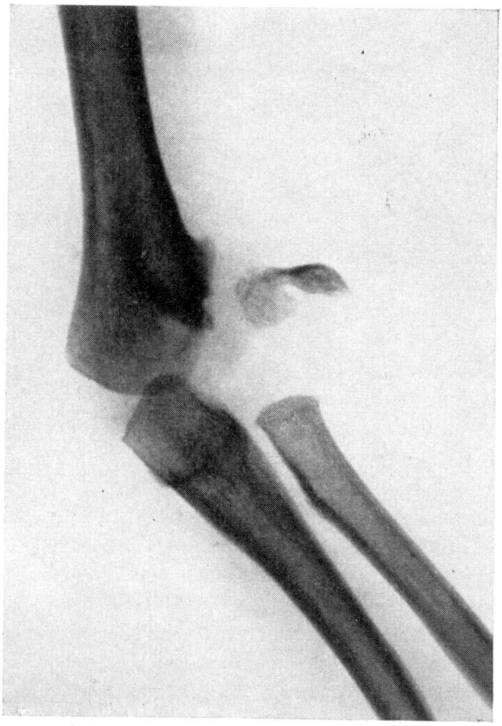

FIG. 56. D. K., male, age 3. Unrecognized fracture of the lateral condyle of two years' duration. There were no subjective symptoms. Slight deformity of the elbow. Treatment not indicated until the child is full grown. (Courtesy Dr. Paul J. Collopy.) [Reproduced with permission of the American Academy of Orthopaedic Surgeons, Instructional Course Lectures (35).]

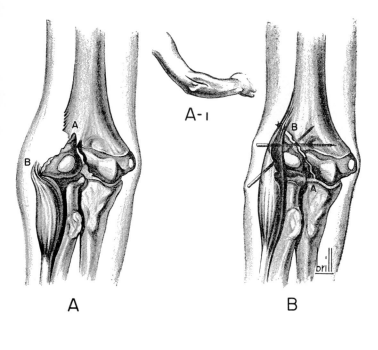

A   B

FIG. 57. A. Diagramatic representation of fracture of the lateral condyle. The extensor muscles of the forearm have rotated the fractured surface A–B laterally and downward through an arc of 90°. The osseous centers of the capitellum and the medial epicondyle are shown in white. A-1. Open reduction is performed through the Kocher lateral incision. B. The rotated lateral condylar fragment has been cleaned of blood clots and pulled back into position with small bone hooks. The fractured surface, A–B, has its normal position. The fragment is fixed with two small pins which are allowed to protrude slightly under the skin. The aponeurosis of the extensor muscles is sutured. [Reproduced with permission of the Journal of the American Medical Association (45).]

FIG. 58. J. B., male, age 4, 7/1/33. Typical lateral condylar fracture with 90° rotation of the fragment in the frontal plane.

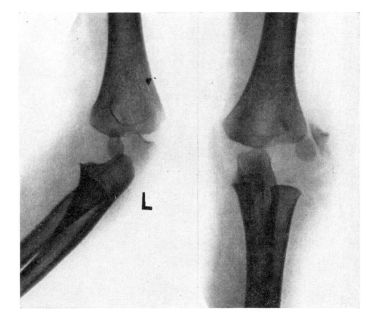

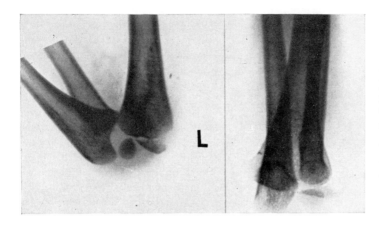

FIG. 59. J. B., 7/1/33. Immediate closed reduction with fair position which was well maintained in the subsequent roentgenograms. The distal fragment of such a fracture frequently displaces within the first two or three days after reduction. Frequent roentgenograms are necessary.

FIG. 60. J. B., 8/2/37. The case shown in the preceding roentgenograms four years after reduction showing persistent enlargement of the left lateral condyle but no change in the carrying angle and no limitarion of elbow motion. Note the trecocious development of the left padial head.

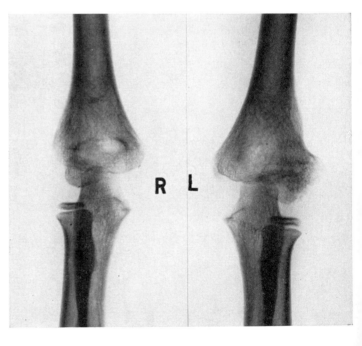

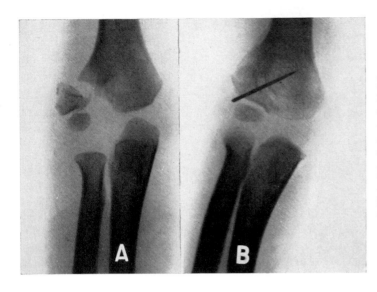

FIG. 61. A. K. L., male, age 3½. Displaced right lateral condylar fracture without much rotation. Open reduction was delayed two weeks because of illness. B. Three weeks after accurate open reduction. The carrying angle was normal. [Reproduced with permission of the American Academy of Orthopaedic Surgeons, Instructional Course Lectures (35).]

FIG. 62. K. L., two and one-half years after the preceding roentgenogram. Solid healing has been accompanied by accelerated longitudinal growth, enlargement of the right lateral condyle, and irregularity of contour. The carrying angle was diminished. Note the precocious maturity of the radial head. There was bony enlargement of the lateral condyle on clinical examination. [Reproduced with permission of the American Academy of Orthopedic Surgeons, Instructional Course Lectures (35).]

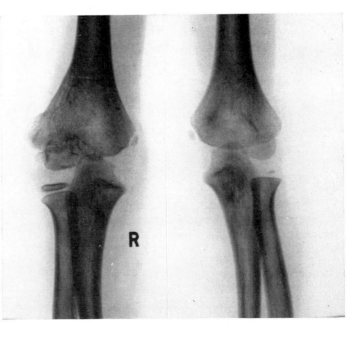

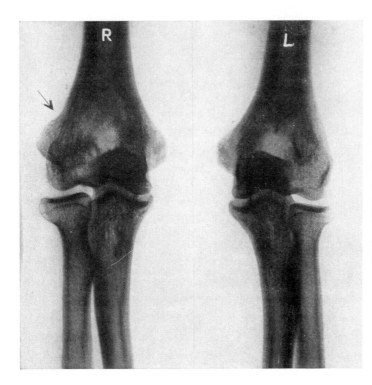

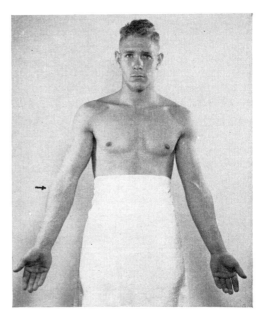

FIG. 64. K. L. Photograph fifteen years following open reduction shows persistent loss of the carrying angle. Elbow motions are normal.

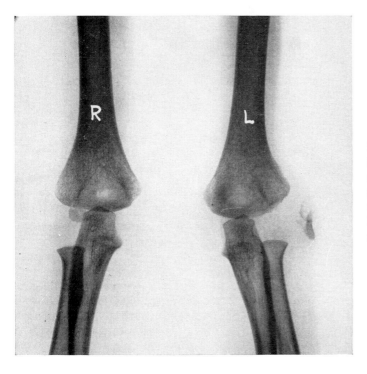

FIG. 65. J. S., male, age 10½, 1/17/50. Three and one-half months following a fracture of the left lateral condyle when the patient fell from a wagon. There was bony enlargement of the lateral condyle of the humerus. Elbow motions were symmetrical.

FIG. 66. J. S., 1/27/50. Open reduction was difficult four months after the injury. Cast applied. Sutures and pin removed four weeks later.

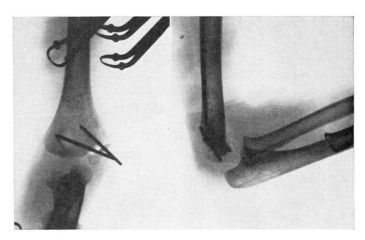

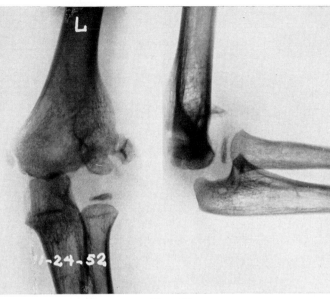

FIG. 67

FIG. 68

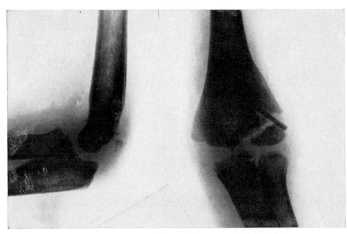

FIG. 69

FIG. 67. J. S. Anteroposterior and lateral views of the left elbow in Figure 66 show solid union but irregularity of the bony contours. Elbow flexion limited 10°. Other motions normal. Clinical examination one year later showed 12° increase in the carrying angle. Motions still the same.

FIG. 68. A. N., male, age 7, 8/12/37. Admitted to the Hospital for Special Surgery on 8/11/37 with an eight week old medial dislocation of the radius and ulna on the humerus with a fracture of the lateral condyle of the humerus (see case A. S., Figure 53). An open reduction was performed on 8/14/37, two months after the injury. Through a posterior incision the soft tissues were completely stripped from the bones. It was necessary to free the proximal fourth of the ulna. The lateral condylar fragment was removed, cleaned of callus and replaced. It was held in position with a beef bone peg. A plaster cast was applied until 8/24/37. (Courtesy of Dr. T. Campbell Thompson.)

FIG. 69. A. N., 11/27/37. The elbow in Figure 68 fourteen weeks postoperative. The capitellar fragment failed to unite, with gradual increase in the carrying angle. Fifteen years later function was excellent with extension 150° and flexion 25°. He was able to play football and baseball and had no complaint. Transplantation of the ulnar nerve may still be necessary. (Courtesy of Dr. T. Campbell Thompson.)

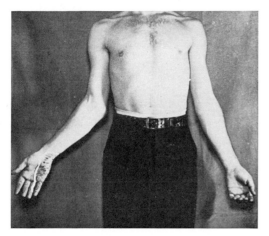

FIG. 70. R. S., male, age 21, 4/13/37. The right lateral condyle was fractured but untreated at age 2. Limitation of elbow motion and pain appeared gradually. Hypesthesia of the ulnar distribution was discovered on examination. [Reproduced with permission of the American Academy of Orthopaedic Surgeons, Instructional Course Lectures (35).]

FIG. 71. R. S., 4/13/37. Anteroposterior roentgenogram of the right elbow shown in the preceding photograph. There was a nonunion of the lateral condyle with upward riding, failure of longitudinal growth on the lateral side and increase in the carrying angle. The acute angulation of the bone had begun to traumatize the ulnar nerve. [Reproduced with permission of the Journal of the American Medical Association (45).]

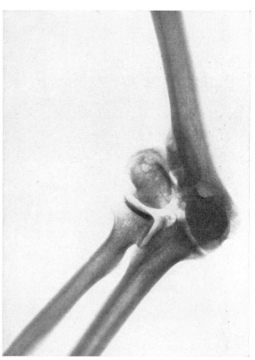

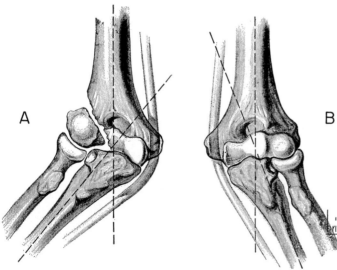

FIG. 72. (A) Schematic representation of nonunion of the right lateral humeral condyle with increase in the carrying angle. Compare with the normal side (B). Prolonged trauma to the ulnar nerve results in the characteristic picture of delayed ulnar nerve palsy. [Reproduced with permission of the Journal of the American Medical Association (45).]

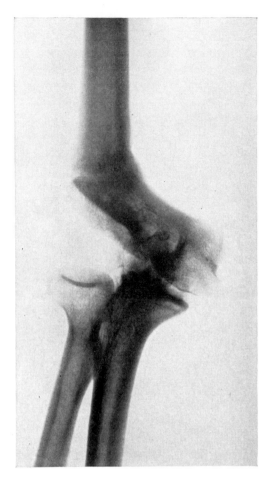

FIG. 73. R. S., 10/8/37. Anteroposterior roentgenogram six months after the deformity in Figure 71 was corrected by osteotomy and the loose fragment removed. Pain was relieved. The hypesthesia over the ulnar distribution disappeared without transplantation of the ulnar nerve. [Reproduced with permission of the American Academy of Orthopaedic Surgeons, Instructional Course Lectures (35).]

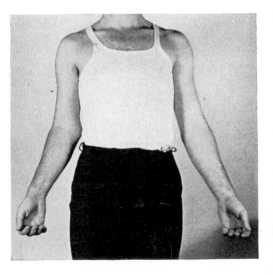

FIG. 74. R. S., 12/1/37, photograph six months following the osteotomy. The carrying angle is now normal on the right. There is still slight limitation of flexion and extension. [Reproduced with permission of the American Academy of Orthopaedic Surgeons, Instructional Course Lectures (35).]

FRACTURES OF THE MEDIAL EPICONDYLE
(8 per cent of elbow fractures)

Medial epicondylar avulsion is the result of sudden valgus strain of the elbow with or without dislocation of the elbow joint. The fragment is an apophysis and not an epiphysis, and takes no part in longitudinal growth. If it is displaced no more than a few millimeters (Fig. 75), the aponeurosis fo the flexor muscles is not completely torn. Brief immobilization in flexion is all that is necessary. Bony healing will usually take place without deformity or disability. If the displacement is greater than five millimeters, one must decide between leaving the fragment displaced or opening the fracture and pinning the fragment in its normal position. Attempts at closed reduction are futile. If the displacement is allowed to persist, nonunion is the rule. Usually there is slight deformity but no disability. In girls this may be more desirable than a scar. Occasionally the displaced fragment is reunited to the metaphysis by a hornlike bony projection.

With marked displacement of the epicondyle there may be prolonged flexion deformity with permanent weakness of elbow flexion. If the injury is diagnosed promptly and there is no contraindication to surgery, open replacement is the procedure of choice in a male. There are only two urgent indications for operation. First, if there are symptoms of ulnar nerve injury, the nerve must be explored promptly and the fracture can be dealt with at the same time. Second, a temporary dislocation of the elbow joint not infrequently leaves the bone fragment incarcerated in the elbow joint (Fig. 76). While it is occasionally possible to angulate the elbow into valgus under anesthesia and pop the fragment out again, there is the danger of causing or aggravating ulnar nerve injury (29). After twenty-four hours, such a manipulation is futile and open operation is indicated (Fig. 77).

When the surgery is performed within a few days of the injury (Fig. 78), the fragment should be pinned back in position (Fig. 79). The ulnar nerve is usually not exposed and may be left in the groove unless preoperative findings suggest exploration. The elbow should be immobilized in plaster at a right angle for four weeks postoperatively as described for lateral condylar fractures. It is well to remove the pins and stitches through a window a week earlier.

If operation is delayed until two weeks after the injury, it is better to excise the bony fragment and suture the aponeurosis of the flexor muscles of the forearm as near their normal position as possible. The loss of the apophysis has no significant effect upon the future development of the elbow. Prompt open reduction uniformly gives an excellent result. If operation is delayed as long as four weeks, prolonged or permanent flexion deformity may occur. After that interval, conservative treatment is usually better. After a delay as long as three months (30), even if the fragment has caught in the elbow joint, the prognosis is better with masterly neglect than with operation.

Medial condylar fractures are exceedingly rare in children (Fig. 81). If they cannot be reduced by manipulation, an operation should be performed promptly (31). Ashhurst (1) made this observation about a case of his in 1910.

COMMINUTED CONDYLAR FRACTURES

"T" fractures and comminuted fractures of the lower end of the humerus, which are common in adults are very rare in children (Fig. 82). Open reductions are frequently necessary in adults and they are notoriously difficult. In children, such operations are rarely justified. Permanent limitation of motion is the rule following ill-advised surgery. If the fracture is seen promptly it may be reduced with surprising accuracy by closed manipulation. With traction in right angle flexion, the fragments are molded into good position and held there by the capsule which is kept taut by the traction of a hanging cast (Fig. 13) for four to five weeks. Temporary limitation of motion following removal of the plaster is treated by masterly neglect (Fig. 84).

FRACTURES OF THE RADIAL NECK
(4.5 per cent of elbow fractures)

The longitudinal thrust that produces a compression fracture of the radial head in an adult causes a fracture of the radial neck in a young child (Fig. 86). Characteristically the buttonlike osseous center with a thin flake of metaphysis is broken off transversely, displaced and angulated radially. If the fracture is incomplete with minimal angulation, no reduction is necessary. If the displacement is partial so that there is some apposition and the angulation is 60° or less, one may manipulate a fresh fracture by angulating the elbow into varus (Fig. 85) and pushing the radial head into improved position. Then the treatment should be conservative (Fig. 87). A cast is applied with the elbow flexed to 90° or somewhat more acutely.

With angulation less than 45°, the end result will be surprisingly good. There is frequently some limitation of supination, but the patient is rarely aware of this. For a period of several months all motions are greatly restricted. The temptation is great to excise the radial head in order to increase the range of motion. While the immediate effect of such an operation is favorable, the late results are tragic (Fig. 88). In the cases that have been followed for several years (32), there has been gross deformity with radial deviation of the hand, shortening of the forearm, increase in the carrying angle, and weakness. *Never excise the radial head in a growing child.*

If the radial head is angulated nearly 90° and displaced so that its fractured surface lies against the shaft (Fig. 89), closed reduction is rarely successful, and prompt open reduction is the treatment of choice. If the operation is performed in the first few days, the immediate and late results should be excellent (Fig. 90). A bad prognosis (33) is not justified (Figs. 91, 92). Great care should be used in handling the epiphysis. It should be gently cleaned of clots and spicules, and pulled into position with small hooks. When the fracture and the radiohumeral dislocation are accurately reduced and the elbow flexed, rotation of the forearm will not displace the fragment. The flexed position should be maintained while the wound is closed and plaster applied. Internal fixation is undesirable and usually unnecessary (34).

If the operative reduction is delayed for a week or two or if the fracture is comminuted, there will be considerable new bone formed and motion will be greatly restricted. As in cases of traumatic myositis ossificans, the treatment should be conservative. Satisfactory motion will gradually return in most cases. Physiotherapy is contraindicated. After three weeks, gross deformity is preferable to an open reduction (35).

Fracture of the radial neck associated with dislocation of the ulno-humeral joint is likely to cause permanent limitation of motion due to the initial soft tissue injury (Figs. 93, 94). In such a case, with persistent restriction of radiohumeral motion, or in the rare fracture of the head of the radius (Fig. 95), operative resection of the head is indicated but should be postponed until the child is almost full grown.

DISLOCATIONS OF THE ELBOW
(6 per cent of elbow injuries)

Dislocation of the elbow joint without fracture is more common in children than in adults. If seen promptly, it is usually reduced with ease by simple traction with the elbow at right angle flexion. If adequate treatment is delayed a week or two, open reduction may be necessary. Ancient dislocations (several months) are best let alone (Fig. 96). The historic pseudoreduction of Robert Jones (20) by manipulating under anesthesia may be helpful in restoring partial flexion, if the elbow is extended.

A three month old dislocation of the radial head in a child either with or without associated fracture should not be reduced by open operation. This dislocation causes little or no disability although it may be unsightly (Fig. 104). It is amazing what good function may prevail with an old untreated dislocation of the radial head. Delayed open reduction re-

sults in permanent limitation of motion. Excision of the radial head in a
child causes the deformity and disability that were discussed under radial
head fractures (Fig. 88) (36). After the child is fully grown, the radial
head may be excised if there is an indication.

Miscellaneous Elbow Injuries

Olecranon fractures occur rarely as isolated injuries in children. Plaster
fixation in extension is the treatment of choice (Fig. 97). Immobilization
for five weeks or longer causes no prolonged or permanent stiffness in a
child as it does in the adult. Ordinary unguided activity soon restores
normal motion. Physical therapy is contraindicated.

Nonunion is not likely in the olecranon fracture of a child. Partite olecranon (patella cubiti) (37) is a developmental anomaly which has been
described erroneously as an ununited fracture in childhood (Fig. 98).
Patella cubiti is usually, but not always, bilateral.

Not infrequently, an olecranon fracture is associated with a fracture of
the radial neck or dislocation of the radial head (Fig. 99). If both are
treated promptly, closed reduction is usually successful. Open reduction
of a dislocated radial head may be necessary particularly after several
day's delay. The Boyd incision (38) gives the best exposure.

Monteggia fractures of the proximal third of the ulna associated with
dislocation of the radial head in children (Figs. 100, 101) can usually be
reduced by closed manipulation (39). When open operation is necessary
in order to reduce the radial head, most often because of delay, internal
fixation of the ulna which is routine in adults (40), is usually superfluous
in children. When the radial head has been reduced by manipulation or by
open operation, the radius usually splints the ulna efficiently (Fig. 102)
If the fracture of the ulna is found to be grossly unstable at the time of
operation it may be fixed by an intramedullary pin inserted through the
olecranon. This should be removed through a window in the cast after
three weeks and the cast left on for a fortnight longer.

Malunited and unreduced Monteggia fractures that are three months
old should be allowed to go untreated. The adaptation of a child to this
situation is remarkable (Fig. 103). A normal range of motion usually develops in spite of the unsightly hypermobility of the radial head (Fig.
104). The latter can be corrected by excision after the child is full grown
without jeopardizing elbow motion. A dislocated radial head should not
be removed. Although not in apposition with the capitellum, it does, nonetheless, press on the soft tissues with the force necessary to promote normal growth. Do not remove the radial head in a growing child.

Subluxation of the radial head under the annular ligament (pulled elbow,
nursemaid's elbow) is a frequent injury in children two to six years old.

At this age the radial head is no greater in diameter than the shaft (41). Although it is accurately described in the early English (42) and French (43, 66) literature in the last century (44) and is well known to pediatrists, this lesion is rarely mentioned in papers on fractures and dislocations (45). It is extremely puzzling to the uninitiated (Fig. 105). The injury is commonly produced by a jerk on the child's upraised arm by the mother who is helping him to step up on a curbstone (Fig. 21, p. 22) or streetcar step (46). It may occur also during rough play with older children or when the arm is caught in the slats of a crib. The subluxation is extremely painful. The elbow is held stiffly in moderate flexion and the forearm in midpronation. The child screams and resists all attempts at help. The roentgenograms are negative. The diagnostic feature is limited supination and pain on any attempted motion.

After an appropriate warning, a deft quick manipulation into supination produces an audible and palpable click associated with sharp pain. Motions then become normal and the pain disappears. The elbow should be immobilized with collar and cuff for a week to prevent recurrence of the subluxation which is not uncommon when support is omitted.

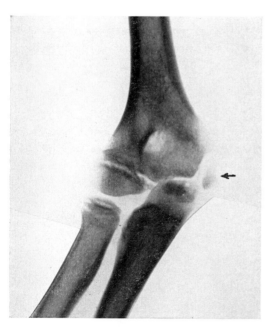

Fig. 75. F. K., male, age 9. Avulsion of the medial epicondyle of the right humerus with minimal displacement. The child recovered completely without treatment other than brief immobilization.

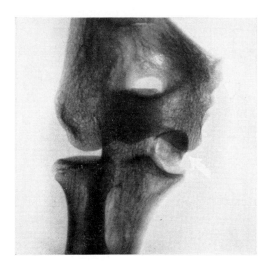

FIG. 76. W. L., male, age 16, 10/14/48. Injury of the right elbow playing football. Immediate pain and swelling with limitation of motion. Open reduction four days later. The medial epicondyle was removed from the elbow joint and pinned in place with two pieces of Kirschner wire. The ulnar nerve was not traumatized and was not disturbed. (Courtesy Dr. Bruce Brewer.)

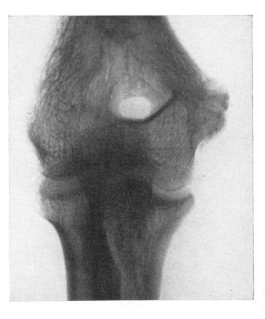

FIG. 77. W. L., 11/12/48. Four weeks following the operation at the time of removal of the pins. Subsequent complete recovery. (Courtesy Dr. Bruce Brewer.)

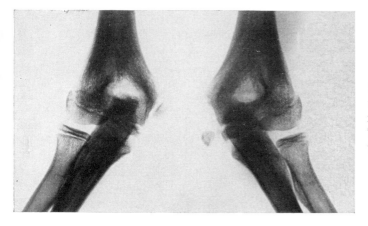

FIG. 78. W. M., male, age 11, 10/24/52. Injury of the left elbow with considerable displacement of the medial epicondyle. Pain and swelling. This degree of displacement was likely to cause permanent disability.

Fig. 79. W. M., 10/28/52. Open reduction and pin fixation of the fracture in Figure 78 four days after the injury.

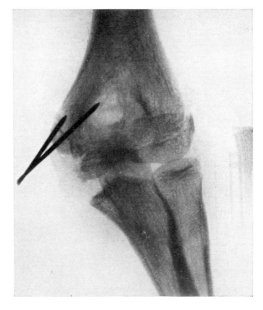

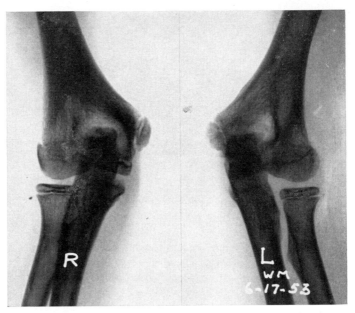

FIG. 80. W. M. Eight months following the open reduction, function is entirely normal.

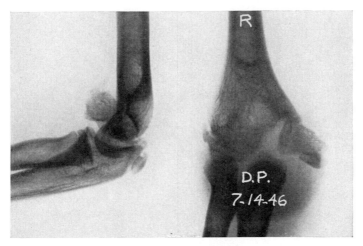

FIG. 81. D. P., male, age 13. Fractured medial condyle of the right humerus when he fell striking his right elbow against a tree stump. The condylar fragment was rotated 90°. Open reduction and fixation with two Kirschner wires on July 16, 1946. Cast and wires removed on August 5, 1946.

Examination two years later

Range of motion at the elbow	Right	Left
Angle of greatest extension	165°	180°
Angle of greatest flexion	35°	25°

Pronation and supination were symmetrical. Right medial condyle slightly prominent. Carrying angles symmetrical. All epiphyses on the right were closed while those on the left were still open (31).

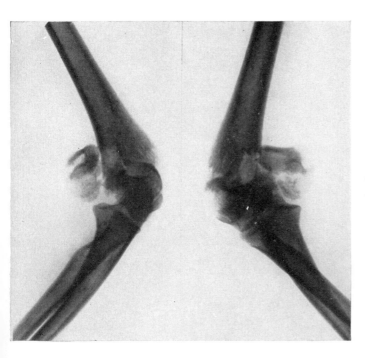

FIG. 82. B. J., female, age 11, 7/27/37. Comminuted condylar fracture of the distal end of the humerus.

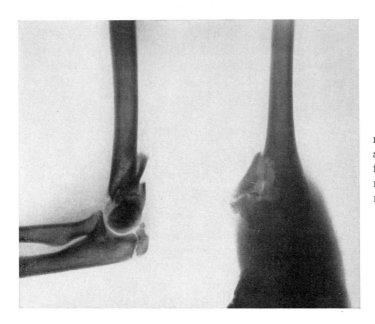

FIG. 83. B. J., 8/29/37. Prompt manipulation under anesthesia and application of a hanging cast secured fair reduction. Roentgenogram on removing the cast. Function rapidly returned to normal.

FIG. 84. B. J., 9/30/38. Fourteen months after the accident, function was normal except for 10° limitation of flexion. This persisted when the patient was examined twelve years after.

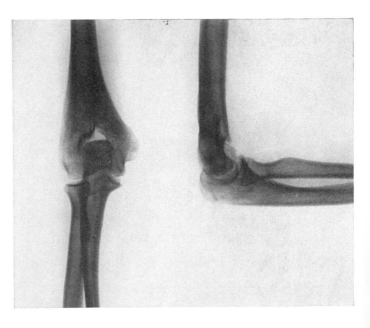

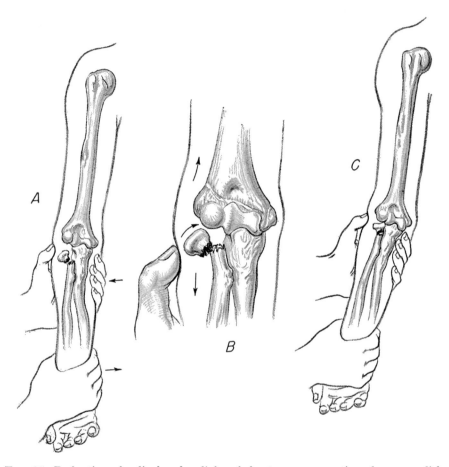

FIG. 85. Reduction of a displaced radial neck fracture can sometimes be accomplished under general anesthesia by angulating the elbow into varus and reducing the fragment with firm digital pressure. With gross displacement, this method is not usually successful.

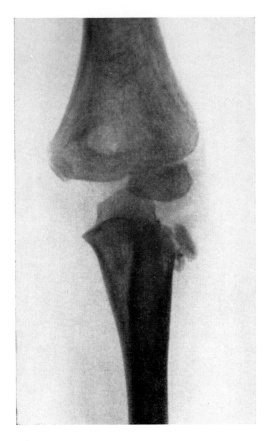

Fig. 86. C. N., female, age 4, 10/19/53. The radial neck was fractured, the epiphyseal fragment was displaced radially and angulated 70° by a fall on the left hand. (Courtesy of Dr. Paul J. Collopy.)

Fig. 87. C. N., 10/19/53. Closed reduction of the fracture in Figure 86 under general anesthesia cut the deformity to 20° of angulation which was acceptable. When examined three months after the injury, all motions were normal except flexion which was limited 15°. Six months later motions were symmetrical. (Courtesy of Dr. Paul J. Collopy.)

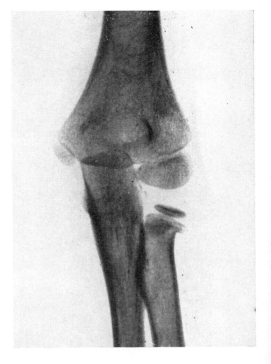

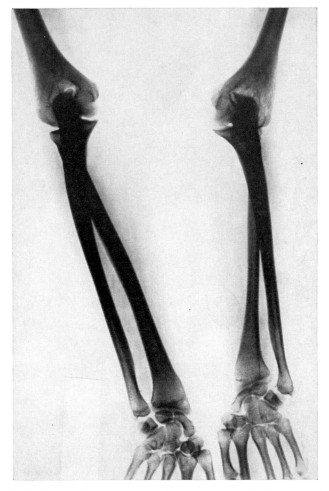

FIG. 88. B. L., female, age 15. Roentgenogram of both forearms nine years after removal of the left radial head for a displaced fracture of the radial neck. The radius was short and delicate. There was radial deviation of the hand and increase in the carrying angle. These deformities were associated with weakness and discomfort. Moral: Never remove the radial head in a growing child. [Reproduced with permission of the Journal of the American Medical Association (52).]

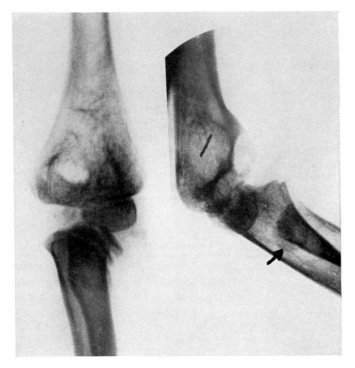

FIG. 89. C. K., female, age 7, 8/13/40. Roentgenogram twenty-four hours after the patient fell on the outstretched left hand. The radial neck was fractured and the head displaced and angulated to the radial side. The arrow points to the radial head in the lateral view.

FIG. 90. C. K., 9/27/40, six weeks after the preceding roentgenogram. On 8/14/40 the left radial head was gently pulled into position with small sharp hooks. No internal fixation was necessary. A molded plaster splint was used to hold the elbow in flexion. The position was maintained with a collar and cuff.

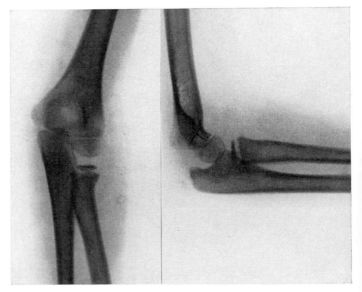

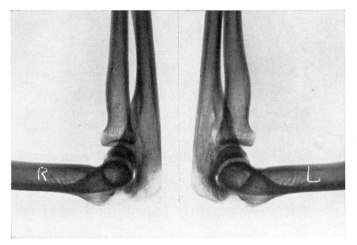

Fig. 91. C. K. Nine years after the fracture, the elbows are radiologically symmetrical except that the left radial neck is slightly thick.

Fig. 92. C. K. In the anteroposterior view the left elbow is normal. Clinically the motions are entirely symmetrical. The carrying angles are the same.

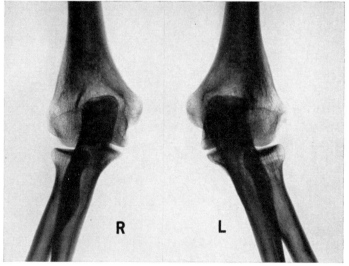

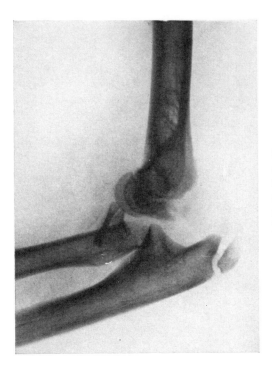

Fig. 93. R. Z., male, age 12, 9/8/48. Fracture of the neck of the radius with dislocation of the elbow and extensive soft tissue injury. Closed reduction of the dislocation. Open reduction of the radial head on the next day. [Reproduced with permission of the American Academy of Orthopedic Surgeons, Instructional Course Lectures (35).]

Fig. 94. R. Z., 2/23/49. Five months after Figure 93 there is excessive new bone formation with very little motion. Resection of the radial head at age sixteen ended in complete ankylosis of the radioulnar joint. Marked restriction of flexion and extension. [Reproduced with permission of the American Academy of Orthopedic Surgeons, Instructional Course Lectures (35).]

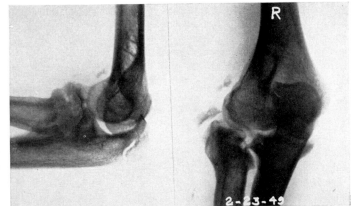

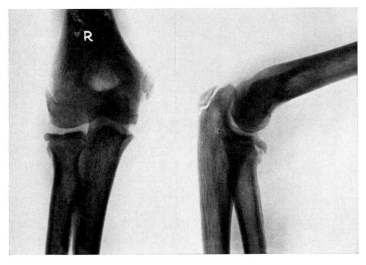

FIG. 95. C. N., male, age 13 Roentgenogram eleven months after a crush injury of the right radial head. Although elbow motions were restricted as follows: extension 40°, flexion 15°, supination 60°, and pronation 20°, he was advised not to have the radial head resected until he was nearly full grown.

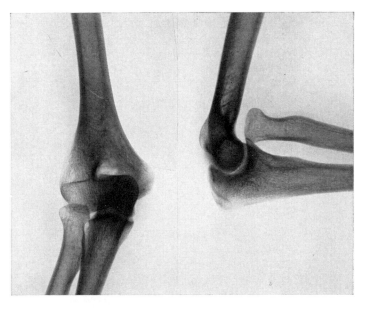

FIG. 96. E. C., female, age 19 The patient did not realize that there was anything wrong with her right elbow until a roentgenogram was taken following a minor accident. The diagnosis of acute dislocation of the radial head was not justified in view of the small atrophic head which had obviously been out of position for many years. Comparison of this plate with one of the opposite elbow would have disclosed at once the abnormal appearance of the right radial head. Moral: Childhood dislocations of the radial head need not be disabling. (Courtesy of Dr. T. Campbell Thompson.)

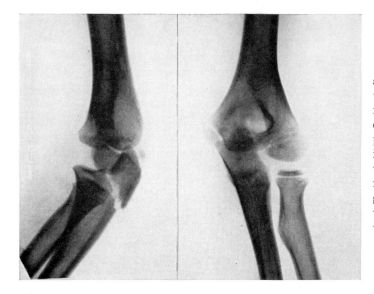

FIG. 97. W. G., 10/18/43, male, age 10, received multiple injuries when he was struck by a car. A roentgenogram revealed a fracture of the olecranon in satisfactory position. The left elbow was splinted in extension. When examined six weeks later the left elbow had normal motion. Checkup roentgenograms four years later showed no trace of the original injury. Motions were symmetrical.

FIG. 98. F. B., male, age 22. Patella cubiti, a congenital anomaly which should not be confused with a childhood fracture. This case was discovered when trauma to the elbow produced a transverse fracture of the projecting distal process of the abnormal bone. The lesion was not bilateral in this case.

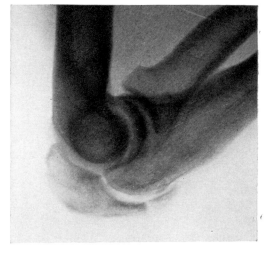

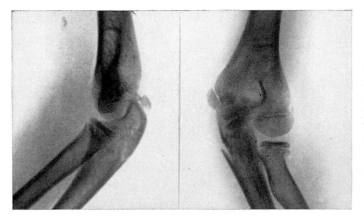

FIG. 99. C. G., female, age 10. Fracture of the olecranon and radial neck without gross displacement. No reduction was necessary. Collar and cuff were worn for three weeks. There were no complications. Examination at one year showed the elbow motions to be normal. The carrying angle was increased 5°.

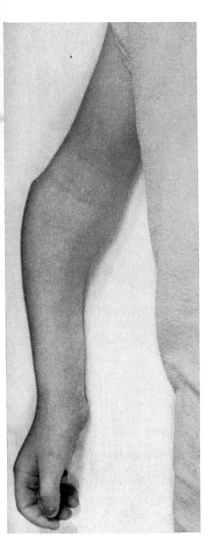

Fig. 100. L. F., female, age 9, 8/14/50. Photograph of a grossly displaced Monteggia fracture of the right elbow (dislocation of the radial head with fracture of the proximal third of the ulna).

Fig. 101. L. F., 8/14/50. Roentgenogram of the preceding displaced Monteggia fracture.

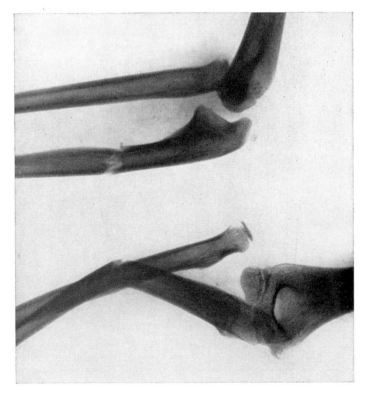

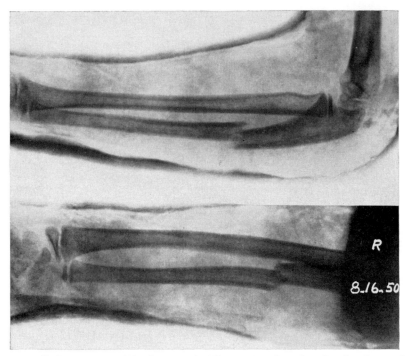

FIG. 102. L. F., 8/16/50. The fracture in Figure 101 after closed reduction and application of a hanging cast. No internal fixation was used. Complete recovery followed. If there is a tendency to displacement of the fracture, an intramedullary pin may be used in the ulna as a temporary measure.

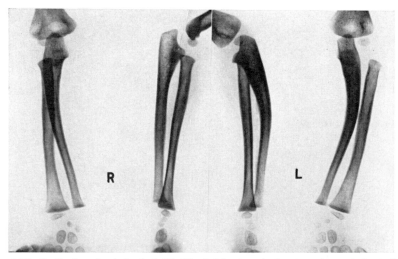

FIG. 103. S. S., female, infant, 6/18/52. A Monteggia fracture in an infant six weeks after the injury. Two views of the left forearm show greenstick angulation of the ulna with displacement of the radial head. The two normals on the right for comparison are absolutely essential in such a case. No treatment. (Courtesy of Dr. A. C. Schmidt.)

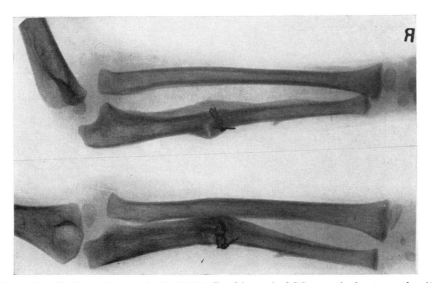

FIG. 104. F. L., male, age 6, 11/28/31. In this typical Monteggia fracture, the dislocated radial head was overlooked and open reduction performed on the ulna two months
before this roentgenogram was taken. Clinical and roentgenographic examination six
years later showed very little change in the ulna, increased displacement of the radial head
but with normal motion and normal function.

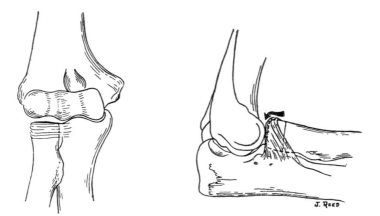

FIG. 105. In a child from two to five years of age, the circumference of the cartilaginous
radial head is the same or smaller than the neck. There is little to keep the annular ligament from subluxating. As shown in the lateral view, the ligament slips between the
capitellum and the radial head when the elbow is hyperextended. By eight years, the
radial head is relatively larger and "pulled" elbow does not occur. [Reproduced with
permission of Magill and Aitken, and Surgery, Gynecology and Obstetrics (41).]

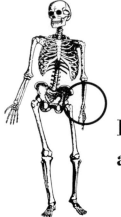

CHAPTER V

Fractures of the Forearm
and Wrist

ETIOLOGY

Fractures of the forearm occur in order of frequency in the distal third (75 per cent), the middle third (18 per cent), and the proximal third (7 per cent). *At the distal end,* they are commonly produced by indirect force from a fall on the hyperextended outstretched hand. The force is the same as that which produces a Colles' fracture in an adult. In a child the roentgenographic appearance varies with the age. In young children there is usually a both bone fracture, frequently greenstick, 1 cm. above the wrist (Fig. 106). From six to twelve, a both bone fracture is likely to be a little higher, with displacement of the distal fragments dorsally (Fig. 107). At this age, the fracture may involve the distal epiphyses with partial or complete displacement.

Fractures of the middle third may be produced by direct or indirect trauma. A direct injury may fracture the radius without the ulna, or the ulna alone. Fracture of one or both bones is likely to be "greenstick" in children and angulated with the apex volar, producing a characteristic deformity (Fig. 108). The mechanics of the *proximal third fractures* are complex, like those of elbow joint injuries.

TREATMENT

The treatment varies with the level of the fracture. Open operation is almost never justified unless the radial head is also dislocated. *Greenstick fractures of the distal third* may be left unreduced if the angulation is not great (Fig. 108). The younger the child and the nearer the fracture is to the end of the bone, the more angulation one may leave unreduced. One should not ordinarily accept more than 30° even in an infant, and this would be excessive in a child of six (Fig. 109). With growth and molding even greater angulation will eventually disappear (Fig. 110). At six or seven, a 30° angle will produce a crooked arm for several months. The parents should be informed that the forearm will be bent at first, but will be perfectly straight eventually.

The closed reduction of a *displaced fracture of both bones of the distal third* of the forearm may require considerable skill. After a delay of a few days it may be impossible. It should be accomplished in the fresh case as follows:

The patient's hand is grasped in one of the surgeons, palm to palm, with the thumb over the dorsum of the distal fragment. The other hand grasps the forearm in symmetrical position with the thumb just above the fracture. The forearm is then angulated as much as 90° with the apex volarward at the same time that strong traction is applied (Fig. 111). This is possible with both thumbs as a fulcrum. The proximal thumb slips down to make firm pressure on the distal fragment of the radius while the operator's other hand straightens out the alignment. Usually both bones can be reduced simultaneously. Checkup roentgenograms should be taken immediately in two planes. Do not use a fluoroscopic examination. It leaves no permanent record—only a permanent effect on the tissues of the surgeon's hands.

If one bone is reduced and the other not, the reduced bone can be used as a lever to distract the unreduced one which is then slipped into position by simple manipulation with the forearm straight. If two or three attempts at closed reduction fail, there may be muscle interposed (Fig. 112). This is not an indication for open operation (Fig. 113). Fixed traction should be applied (Figs. 114, 115). The result will be a functionally normal forearm within six months (Figs. 116, 118) and normal bone architecture on roentgenographic examination within eighteen months in a child of about six years (Fig. 118).

A fracture of the radius alone or of both bones at the distal end should be reduced in full pronation (66) unless the fragments stay reduced better with somewhat less pronation and immobilized in a cast extending above the flexed elbow (Fig. 119). A circular plaster is better than splints. The wrist should be in neutral flexion. Molding under the volar aspect of the radius to accentuate the normal curve, is more effective than forced volar flexion of the wrist (52) in maintaining reduction. Pronation will relax the pronator quadratus and by twisting the radius "around the ulna", overcome the strong tendency to recurrence of the angulation with the apex volarward.

The cast should extend distally to the knuckles. In a child there is no need to permit free flexion of the metacarpophalangeal joints. Fingers do not become stiff following five weeks of partial immobilization. The hand portion of the cast will be battered to pieces with loss of position if one is too careful about freeing the child's hand.

Following reduction and the application of a cast, a roentgenogram that shows satisfactory alignment while the patient is asleep, must be repeated in a few days to prove that angulation has not occurred from muscle pull. Another plate should be taken in two weeks. It is better to discover angulation in time to correct it easily than to find it when the cast is removed (Figs. 120–122). Fragments that remain in malposition can be refractured at five weeks but it is much easier at two (Fig. 123).

Bayonet apposition in good alignment is not to be confused with angular deformity. The side to side contact produces no deformity or limitation of motion and is acceptable. Healing is solid in less time than with end to end apposition. Slight enlargement of the wrist rapidly disappears. Length should not be a problem. If there is appreciable overriding, it should be corrected and the position maintained with traction. When there is no tendency to displacement, there is no objection to midrotation. The wrist should be in neutral flexion (Fig. 119), slight palmar flexion rather than dorsiextension as advised in fractures of the hand. Extreme volar flexion of the wrist is awkward.

Occasionally it is permissible to cut the cast and wedge it but care must be used to avoid harmful pressure. Pressure pads or pressure rods between the bones are not necessary in children and should be avoided because of the danger of ischemic necrosis. Casts must be split and spread, or bivalved if there is any threat to the circulation.

Too many men treat roentgenograms instead of children. I have been asked frequently how I satisfy parents who wish to see the roentgenogram which looks like Figure 117. The formula is simple. I bring out a set of roentgenograms which I keep in readiness which look even worse than the case under treatment. I show how the deformed bone returns rapidly to normal appearance. The gratitude of the parents at the end of treatment is worth the trouble expended in explaining the prognosis.

Many of my colleagues who have taken the easy course and replaced the fragments in anatomic position by open operation have confessed to various complications. Nonunion is all too frequent (5). Several cases of pseudarthrosis at the distal end of the radius requiring bone graft have been reported by personal communications. There are several reports in the literature (47, 48, 49). Delayed union is common following operation. Deformity due to unequal growth is not uncommon (Figs. 124–126). Infection cannot be ignored. The scar is objectionable in a girl. Disastrous complications are rare but they are inexcusable when the results with closed methods are so good (51).

A *reverse distal forearm fracture* in which the force is applied with the wrist in volar flexion, is somewhat more frequent in children than in adults, among whom it almost disappeared with the automobile crank.

It occurs in children who fall on the back of the volar flexed hand. When the fracture is displaced, reduction is usually easy. This fracture should be put up in some degree of dorsiextension.

Fractures of the middle third of the forearm should not be allowed to remain angulated to any appreciable degree except in very young children. Reduction may be carried out as described for the distal third, usually with the forearm in midrotation. An angulation or rotation deformity here will persist for years (in older children, permanently) and limit pronation and/or supination (66). A true estimate of the amount of angulation frequently necessitates accurate roentgenograms of both forearms in symmetrical positions and several projections. The normal curves of the bones are deceiving.

Greenstick fractures at this level (Figs. 127–129) as recommended by Malgaigne (65) should be broken completely through by a quick, deft bending force over the surgeon's knee (Fig. 130), (not "jerking, uncontrolled movement") (50). Anesthesia is not required in a fresh case. After the fractures have been completed with an audible snap, the fragments will remain in good position while the forearm is suspended by the fingers and a plaster case applied from the knuckles to midarm with the elbow at a right angle and the forearm in midrotation. There is no tendency to displacement. Cross union has not occurred in our series, and I have never heard of a verified case (66). If a greenstick fracture is not broken through but merely bent to the straight position as advocated by some (50), the deformity will usually recur within the cast. Wedging of the cast or the use of a pressure pad to prevent the return of deformity (50) is an invitation to Volkmann's ischemia. The appearance of pain is a danger signal here as it is at the elbow.

The position of a fracture of the middle third can be maintained by a simple cast (Fig. 131) with neutral version in most cases. Loss of alignment is no indication for open reduction. Satisfactory position can be restored with skin traction applied to the fingers with rubber bands (Fig. 115) over a banjo wire incorporated in the conventional arm cast with the elbow at a right angle and the forearm in midrotation (Fig. 114). There is no risk of stiffness when the fingers of a child are immobilized with traction but the danger associated with open reduction of this fracture cannot be ignored. Apposition is not necessary and 5 mm. of overriding will be equalized by accelerated growth (Figs. 136—138). Nonunion does not occur, even in the absence of treatment. Slight shortening is insignificant in the forearm.

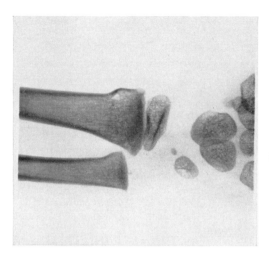

.Fig. 106. R. W., male, age 6. Greenstick (torus) fracture of both bones just above the wrist. Immobilization with a short cast or a splint for two to three weeks relieves the symptoms. Complications do not occur.

Fig. 107. L. T., male, age 11, 1/5/33. Both bone fracture characteristic of the age, 3 to 4 cm. above the wrist joint. Closed reduction failed. The fragments were immobilized in normal alignment with bayonet apposition, dorsal displacement of the distal fragments. Healing was prompt without deformity. A followup study five years later showed normal motion, strength, and appearance. There was no radiologic evidence of fracture.

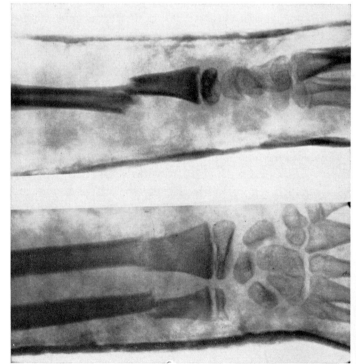

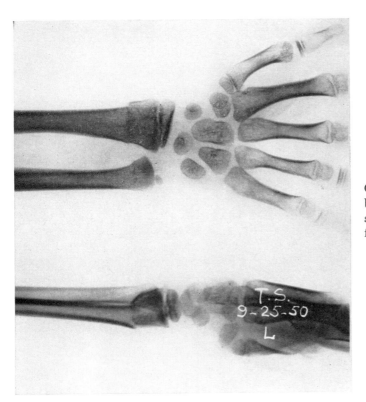

FIG. 108. T. S., female, age 7. Greenstick fracture, distal end, both bones of the forearm. A cast was applied. The patient did not return for five weeks.

FIG. 109. T. S., five weeks after the preceding roentgenogram when the cast was removed. A checkup roentgenogram should have been taken in one week. The child had a bad cold. The angulation of 44° remained. The bowing with the convexity volar was almost gone in six weeks.

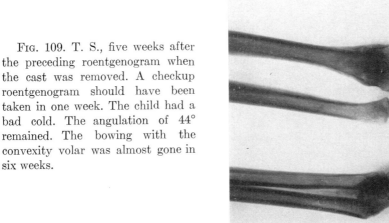

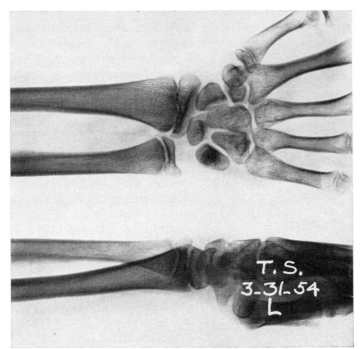

FIG. 110. T. S., followup roentgenograms three and one-half years after the fracture. The left forearm and wrist are clinically and radiologically normal. Moral: Angular deformities in the plane of motion of a joint of a young child straighten out to a remarkable degree.

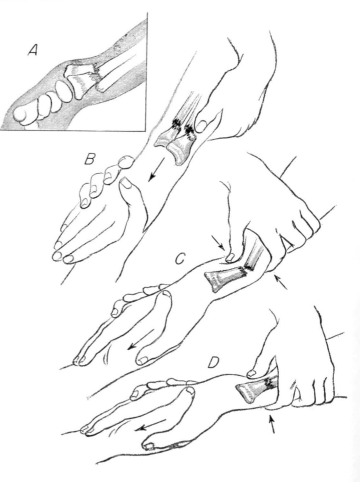

FIG. 111. The displaced both bone fracture of the distal end of the forearm (A) can sometimes be reduced by simple traction and manipulation (B). In the difficult case this is not possible. Then it is well to combine traction with angulation apex volar. One of the examiner's thumbs is used as a fulcrum as shown in (C). The fragments may be angulated as much as 90° if necessary. After the ends are engaged the thumb is slipped down over the distal fragment (D) and the bones are straightened out.

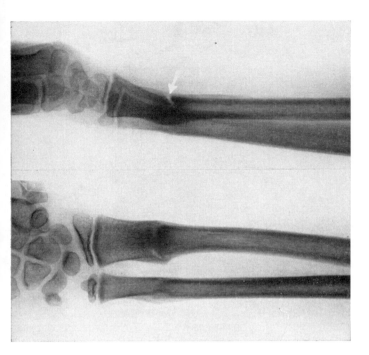

FIG. 112. P. L., female, age 9. A closed both bone fracture of the distal third of the forearm at characteristic level. Muscle tissue had been included between the bone ends as seen in the lateral view. This disappeared within three months. Solid union occurred.

FIG. 113. R. J., male, age 5, 1/28/38, sustained the characteristic forearm fracture for this age when his sled struck a parked car. Following two unsuccessful attempts at closed reduction under anesthesia, alignment was maintained and overriding reduced to a minimum by traction, applied as illustrated in Figure 114. [Reproduced with permission of the Journal of the American Medical Association (52).]

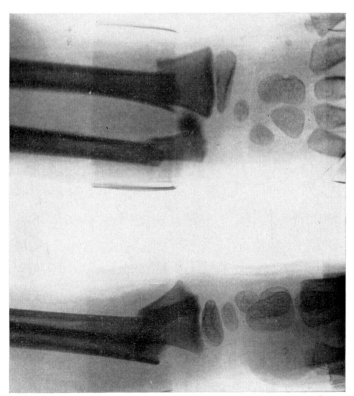

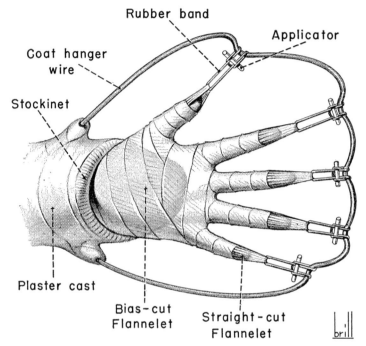

Rubber band

Applicator

Coat hanger
wire

Stockinet

Plaster cast

Bias-cut
Flannelet

Straight-cut
Flannelet

Fig. 114. Skin traction may be used on the fingers of a child (not in an adult) for three weeks or more without ill effect. By this means, the alignment of any forearm fracture may be maintained. Apposition is of no consequence. [Reproduced with permission of Clinical Medicine (143).]

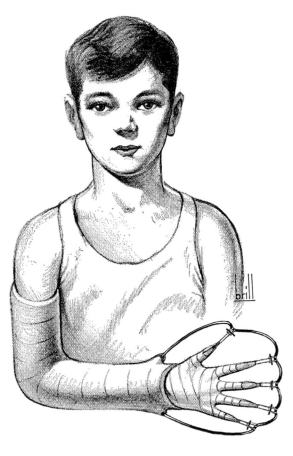

FIG. 115. The banjo traction was attached to a long arm cast with the elbow flexed. This was changed for a long arm cast without traction, seventeen days after the fracture.

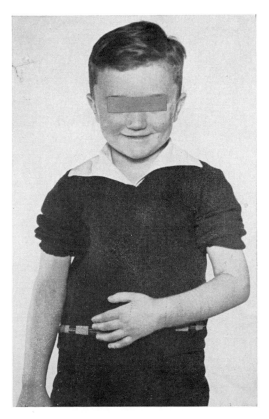

FIG. 116. R. J. Except for slight swelling the appearance of the wrist was normal on removal of the second cast. Clinically normal alignment is important in forearm fractures in children. [Reproduced with permission of the Journal of the American Medical Association (52).]

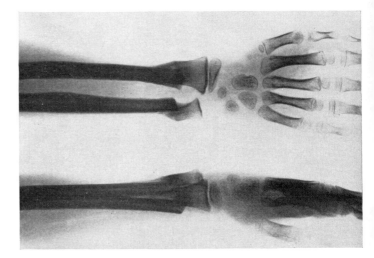

Fig. 117. R. J., 3/4/38. Five weeks following the fracture there was good alignment, solid union, and minimal shortening. [Reproduced with permission of the Journal of the American Medical Association (52).]

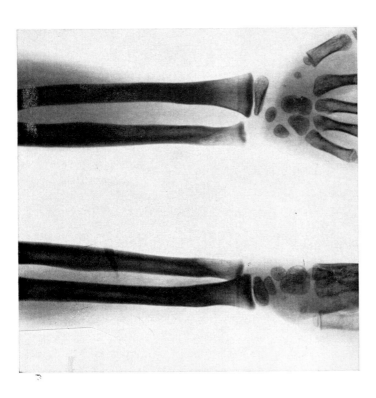

Fig. 118. R. J., 8/19/38. Eight months after the fracture, the roentgenogram shows almost complete restoration of the internal architecture. Clinically the forearm was normal. In the roentgenograms taken eighteen months after the injury, the left looked just like the right. [Reproduced with permission of the Journal of the American Medical Association (52).]

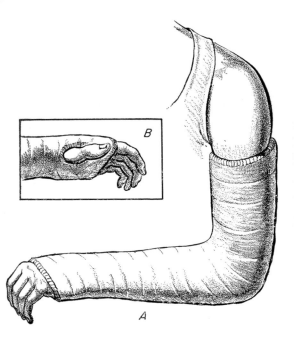

FIG. 119. Fractures of the distal third of the forearm should be immobilized in pronation; slight pronation for fractures of the radius only, and somewhere between mid and full pronation for both bones. In a child, the wrist need not be in the position of function. Extreme palmar flexion serves no useful purpose either. Slight palmar flexion is the neutral position. The cast should be molded under the volar surface of the radius.

FIG. 120. F. Y., male, age 10, 12/29/51. This greenstick fracture of the left radius with a complete fracture of the ulna occurred when the child fell out of a double decker bed breaking the fall with his left hand. It was reduced by a local practitioner who did not break the radius through, but merely bent the forearm straight.

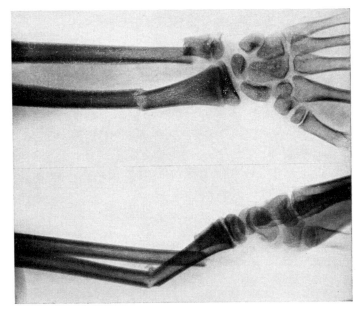

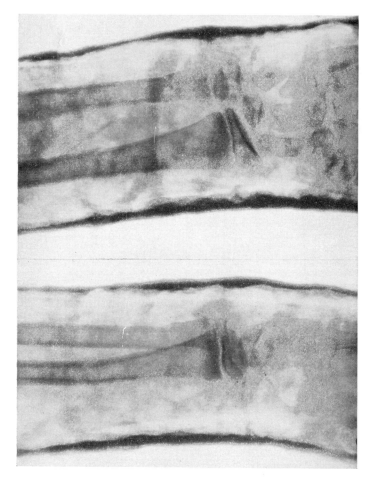

Fig. 121. F. Y. This roentgeno-gram was taken through the cast just after the incomplete reduction, before the patient resumed activity.

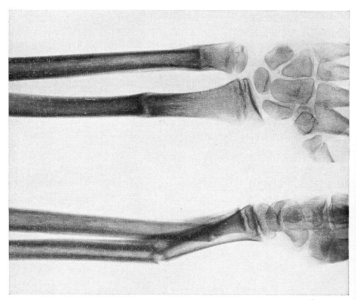

Fig. 122. F. Y. When the cast was removed seven weeks later the deformity had recurred. Pronation was obliterated. In a boy of ten years, with the fracture so near the middle of the bone, and angulated to this degree, the deformity was not acceptable.

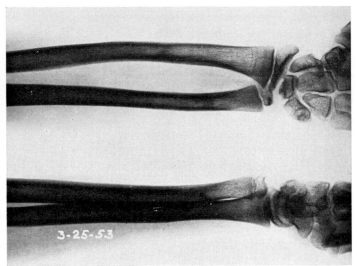

FIG. 123. F. Y., 3/25/53, one year after the preceding film. The arm was refractured on 2/20/52 and put up in marked pronation. The alignment of the radius was restored. The ulna was not refractured. At the end of a year, function was normal. Morals: 1. Angulation of greenstick fractures of the forearm is likely to recur unless the fracture is completed. 2. Fractures of the radius near the distal end are put up in pronation.

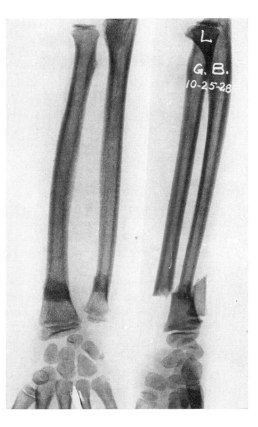

FIG. 124. G. B., female, age 8, 10/25/28. Complete closed fracture of the distal end of the radius. Closed reduction attempted unsuccessfully on two occasions. Open reduction on 11/2/28, one week after the fracture. Discharged from the hospital in a plaster splint.

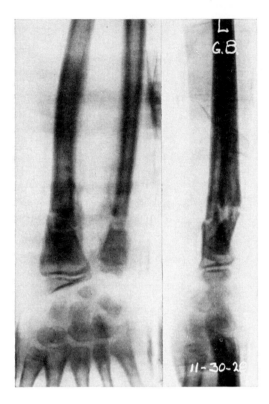

FIG. 125. G. B., 11/30/28. In the plaster splint one month after the fracture. The position of the fragments is satisfactory.

FIG. 126. G. B., 6/30/36, eight years following the fracture. Note that open reduction has "done something" to the left forearm. Following closed reductions, deformity does not occur (compare R. J., Figure 113). There was bowing of both radius and ulna with the convexity laterally. Appreciable shortening of the forearm bones. Sixty degrees of limitation of pronation, 10 of supination. Other motions were normal. Slight loss of the carrying angle. Pain in the wrist with heavy work.

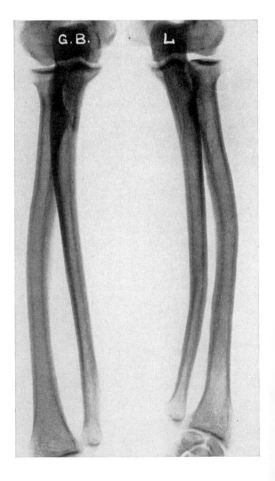

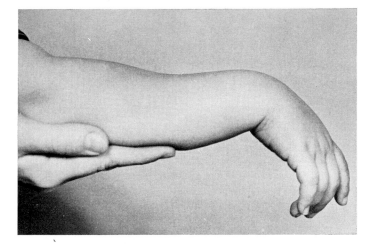

Fig. 127. R. K., male, age 3½, 6/21/47. Typical greenstick fracture of both bones of the forearm. The true angulation is masked by baby fat.

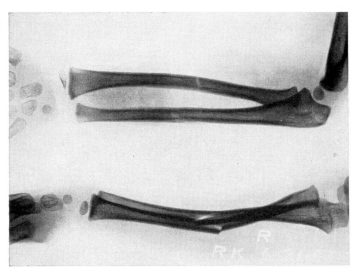

Fig. 128. R. K., 6/21/47. Greenstick both bone fracture of the middle third. Both bones were broken through (Fig. 130) and a long cast was applied with the forearm in midrotation. The soft tissue hinge that Charnley describes (53) is desirable, but a bony bridge will serve as a spring to reproduce the deformity unless it is broken through.

Fig. 129. R. K., 8/1/47, healed fracture shown in the previous roentgenogram six weeks later. Union is solid. The alignment is normal. The ulna normally bows with the convexity dorsally.

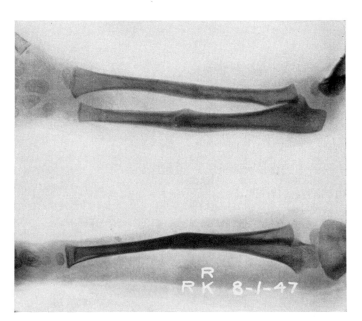

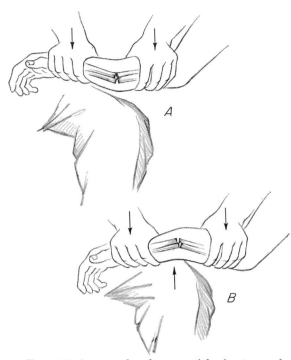

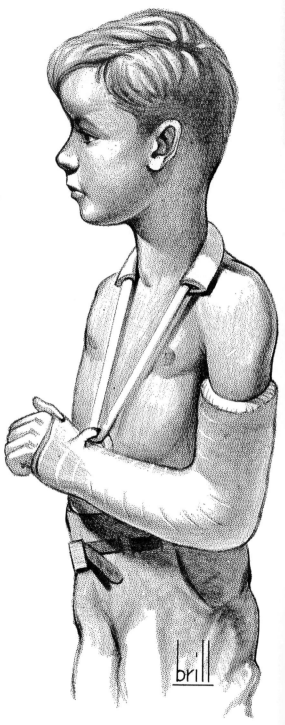

FIG 130. An angulated greenstick fracture of
both bones of the forearm (A) should not almost be
straightened out, but should be broken through by
a deft bending force over the surgeon's knee. (B).
The deformity should be slightly reversed. The
bone is broken but the periosteum remains intact.
Following this maneuver, the forearm will remain
straight while suspended by the fingers. Recurrence
of the deformity does not occur, as it does so often
if the fracture is not completed.

FIG. 131. A long arm cast with the elbow flexed
to 90° and the forearm in neutral version is routine
for fractures of the middle third. It is not necessary
to leave the knuckles free. Immobilization of a
child's finger joints does not cause stiffness unless
there is a hand injury.

Displaced fractures of the proximal third are reduced with the forearm in complete supination (Fig. 132) and held in a plaster cast (Fig. 133). Overriding is not objectionable but alignment must be good (52). If there is a tendency to angulation, it must be corrected by traction applied to the fingers as suggested for fractures of the middle third. Bayonet apposition is acceptable since there will be perfect restoration of the bony contours in a few months and roentgenograms will look normal within a year. Function will be normal. Malposition is an indication for more efficient conservative measures and not for open reduction.

Fractures of a single bone in the forearm at any level offer an interesting problem. If the fragments are displaced appreciably an attempt should be made at reduction. The sound bone may be used as a lever and considerable force exerted in traction on the broken one (Fig. 134). Pronation is useful in maintaining the position of a fracture of the distal end of the radius; supination, of the proximal end. Accurate reduction hastens the return of function. It is not essential (Figs. 137, 138). There will be solid union, even if the bone ends are moderately displaced. Callus will bridge interposed muscle masses in children (Fig. 112). Restricted pronation and supination will eventually return to normal unless there is gross displacement in a boy over twelve (a girl over ten). Only when there is irreducible angulation at the middle third in a child over this age, is open reduction justified. Internal fixation is unnecessary.

Refracture of both bones of the forearm at the same level is more frequent than generally realized (Fig. 135). It usually occurs within the first six months after the original injury, but may be delayed longer. The reason is probably related not to any weakness of the bones, but to the child's habit pattern. Tumbles at a certain age are due to temporary awkwardness or carelessness. When the fall occurs, it is characteristically broken by the outstretched hand that is not carrying a toy. The same trauma is likely to be repeated. After a year or more, other activities cause other injuries.

Epiphyseal Fractures

Epiphyseal fractures of the distal end of the forearm are unique in children and usually occur between the ages of six and ten. The radius alone or both bones may be involved. Sometimes displacement of the radial epiphysis is combined with a greenstick fracture of the ulna. Marked displacement of the epiphyseal fragment is usually produed by direct trauma (Fig. 139).

The diagnosis of a displaced epiphyseal fracture is readily made by the roentgenogram. Occasionally there is spontaneous reduction. Then one should recognize the diagnostic importance of a tiny chip of metaphysis which usually remains attached to the dorsum or radial side of the epiphyseal fragment (3). It is an indication that there had previously been displacement. When seen promptly, the fracture is easily reduced (Fig. 140). As in fractures through the distal end of the shaft, minor displacements need not be reduced. There will be prompt restoration of both function, and form on the roentgenographic film. Slight overgrowth is common but retardation from epiphyseal injury is rare in this type of fracture (Fig. 141).

The slightly displaced fracture through the epiphysis of the radius (Fig. 142) produced indirectly by a fall with considerable force on the outstretched hand may appear insignificant, but the associated crushing injury to the growing cells of the epiphyseal plate is likely to cause retarded epiphyseal growth. Angular deformity appears promptly as the bone elongates (Figs. 143, 144). The prognosis should take this possibility into consideration (Fig. 147). Prompt recognition is important if treatment is to be efficient (Figs. 145, 146). Repeated osteotomies are preferable to early closure of the radial epiphysis to prevent the return of angular deformity. Not more than 5 mm. of elongation should be attempted at one operation. The radial deviation of the hand secondary to epiphyseal fracture of the distal end of the radius must be differentiated from a true Madelung's deformity (Fig. 148), which is usually bilateral, and asymptomatic until puberty.

Epiphyseal fractures are treated like other fractures of the distal end of the forearm. Open reduction is rarely necessary (Figs. 149–151). The end result is influenced less by accuracy of reduction than by the amount of initial trauma to the growing cells of the epiphysis. Forcible or repeated reductions and particularly open reduction of an ephiphyseal fracture which is more than two weeks old should be avoided because of the danger of additional trauma to the epiphyseal plate. After displacement of an epiphysis, realignment takes place subperiosteally and the shaft soon follows the epiphysis to the new position. Apply the same rules for acceptability of the deformity as for both bone fractures above the epiphysis.

Fractures and Dislocations of the Carpus

Injuries of the carpus are exceedingly rare until a child is almost full grown. Fresh dislocations of the semilunar are reduced in the same manner as for adults (54).

Fractures of the carpal scaphoid are usually not displaced. They may be difficult to recognize as in adults. Roentgenograms of both wrists should be taken with the fists clenched in the dorsipalmar projection, and in the oblique position. Reray in a week if the first roentgenogram is negative.

Plaster immobilization including the thumb must be continued until there is roentgenologic evidence of healing. This usually means eight weeks, but it may take six months.

Occasional carpal fractures will benefit by open reduction. Fracture of the carpal semilunar is rarely encountered as an isolated injury. Such a fracture with displacement of one fragment could not be reduced by closed methods (Fig. 152). An associated crushing epiphyseal fracture of the distal end of the radius which was easily reduced by closed methods caused permanent shortening, while the carpal semilunar healed perfectly following open reduction (Figs. 153 to 155).

Ligamentous injuries of the carpus require two weeks of complete immobilization plus one week of splinting with supervised gentle motion at the times of dressing.

WRINGER INJURIES[2]

Etiology

A fracture of the middle third of the forearm, and occasionally at another level in the upper extremity of a child is sometimes the result of a wringer or mangle injury. The fracture may occur at the time of the accident or later as a pathologic fracture following denudation of the bone (Fig. 156). In either case the fracture is of secondary importance. The mechanism of the soft tissue injury should be thoroughly understood if treatment is to be appropriate.

The young child is fascinated by the moving wringer of a semiautomatic washing machine and catches his fingers in the turning rollers if not watched. The wringer overpowers the screaming child and draws part or all of the arm into the machine. At times it may pull a small child off his feet. If the victim is fortunate, someone stops the motor and sets off the safety release. If rescue is delayed, the wringer mechanism will churn the soft parts at either elbow or axilla, damaging severely the underlying muscles, vessels and nerves at this point of injury. This severe "crush injury" is a true surgical emergency and should be handled by someone who is familiar with the proper treatment. Neglect or improper treatment at this time results in further damage.

Examination

The arm may appear completely unharmed or only slightly damaged. A few superficial abrasions, lacerations, ecchymoses, or a moderate amount of edema may be all that is noted. When "churning" has occurred, there is usually a small area of "brush burn" in the antecubital fossa or

---

[2] This section is based upon the pioneer work of Dr. Irwin Schulz of Milwaukee, Wisconsin and is written with his collaboration and the help of Dr. Frackelton.

axilla. It is impossible to estimate the degree of damage at the first examination, since the most serious element of the injury is the progressive tissue destruction that is hidden beneath the skin surface.

Pathologic Changes

In addition to the crushing of underlying muscles, tendons, nerves, and blood vessels, there is hemorrhage into fascial planes, extravasation of blood and tissue fluid. A sleeve of skin and subjacent tissue separates from the underlying fascia shearing off the intervening and connecting vascular plexus. The arm may be compared to a semidenuded musculoskeletal understructure incased in a pedicle graft sleeve. The pedicle graft sleeve has been stretched, twisted, and crushed. Salvage of this damaged sleeve is dependent upon limiting the "white bleeding" of tissue fluid extravasation and pooling of the hematoma and by giving turgor support to tissues to improve their circulation.

Vascular spasm and ischemic necrosis begin soon and may progress to a disastrous degree within twenty-four hours. These changes can be minimized or prevented by proper treatment instituted immediately after the accident. Even after thirty-six hours, progressive damage can be arrested. A poorly handled case may go on to extensive necrosis of muscles, tendons, nerves, and bone (Fig. 156) of the entire limb. Infection may supervene in the damaged tissue. This disaster means complete destruction of tissue that might otherwise have been salvaged.

Ischemic necrosis is the most damaging component of wringer injury. It is preventable if proper treatment is begun early. Hot compresses and strong antiseptics increase tissue loss and should be avoided. Proper treatment stops progressive loss of tissue and salvages structures which have been injured but are still viable.

Treatment

The arm is examined and roentgenograms taken. If there are fractures they are reduced and splinted when the pressure dressing is applied. The the injured extremity is cleansed thoroughly with soap and water under aseptic precautions. Complicated cases are treated in the operating room with the surgeon in cap, mask, gown, and sterile gloves. Anesthesia is used if needed. Superficial and deep lacerations are repaired but not closed tightly. Any large hematomas are evacuated by aspiration. Sterile petrolatum strips are applied lengthwise (not circularly) on the abrasions and repaired lacerations. Several layers of gauze are interposed between the fingers to avoid skin to skin contact. Kerlix roll bandage is wound about the extremity from the fingertips to well above the point of maximum injury. Mechanics' waste has been discarded because it is difficult to apply evenly. A cotton elastic (not rubberized) bandage gives further firm compression. The fingertips are left exposed so that the circulation may be carefully watched. This type of elastic pressure dressing gives support to the damaged vessels by preventing further edema and extravasation.

When a fracture is present, a light plaster cast is applied over the pressure dressing to maintain reduction. The forearm and arm are elevated and surrounded with ice packs. *Never apply heat.* A suitable antibiotic is given in the presence of abrasions and lacerations.

Results

Two end result studies have been made at the Milwaukee Children's Hospital (55, 56), the first of 45 patients in the period from 1935 to 1941 and the second of 114 cases including the first series from 1935 to 1951. Many of the 45 patients (1935 to 1941) were treated late and by inadequate or harmful methods. The application of hot compresses produced the worst results. The other 69 cases (1942 to 1951) showed markedly improved results. This was a reflection of local publicity regarding the seriousness of wringer injury and its proper treatment. The patients in the second group were brought to the hospital earlier; the late ones received better medical care. Skin grafts were necessary in fewer cases (57). The periods of hospitalization were markedly reduced.

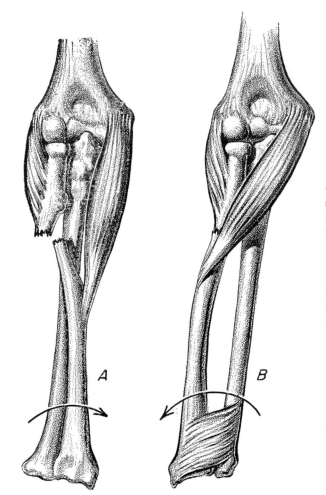

FIG. 132. Fractures of the radius or both bones in the proximal third should be reduced and immobilized in supination. A. The proximal fragment of the radius is controlled by the supinator muscle. B. The distal fragment is influenced by two pronators which must be stretched out by pronating the forearm to align the distal fragment with the proximal.

FIG. 133. A long forearm cast should be applied in supination for fractures of the proximal third. If there is any angulation or excessive overriding, a banjo attachment with skin traction on the fingers may be added (Fig. 115).

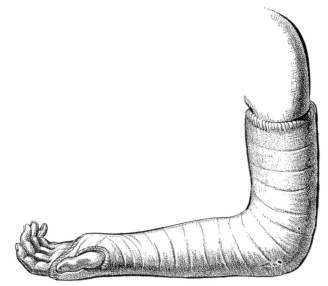

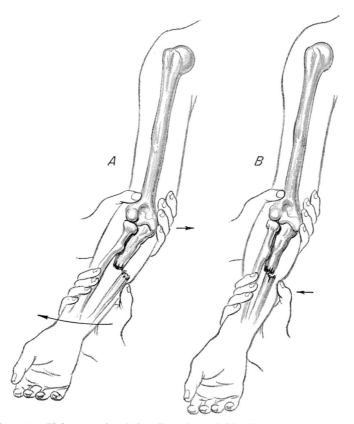

FIG. 134. Valgus strain of the elbow is useful in distracting the radial fragments when only the radius is broken. Traction is less important than the leverage action at the wrist (A) by using the ulna as a fulcrum. B. The distal fragment is manipulated into position with the thumb.

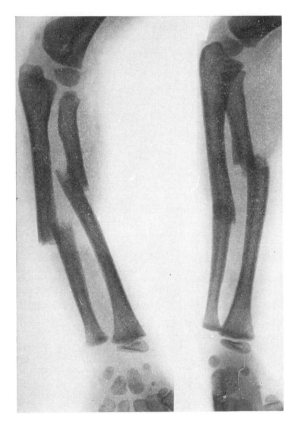

FIG. 135. L. B., male, age 6, 1/4/36. Refracture of both bones at the site of a greenstick fracture of both bones three and one-half months previously. Good alignment but no apposition was obtained in a simple cast. [Reproduced with permission of the Journal of the American Medical Association (52).]

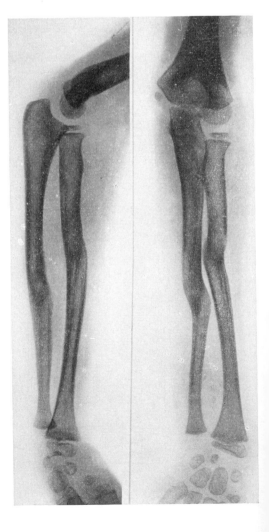

FIG. 136. L. B., 7/22/36, six months after the preceding film. Union had occurred with good alignment. There was still slight limitation of pronation. This disappeared within three months. [Reproduced with permission of the Journal of the American Medical Association (52).]

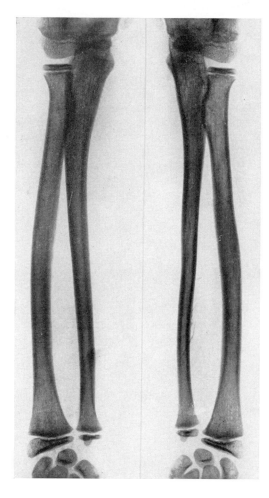

FIG. 137. L. B., 11/8/40, five years after the original injury. There was no radiologic evidence of the fracture. [Reproduced with permission of the Journal of the American Medical Association (52).]

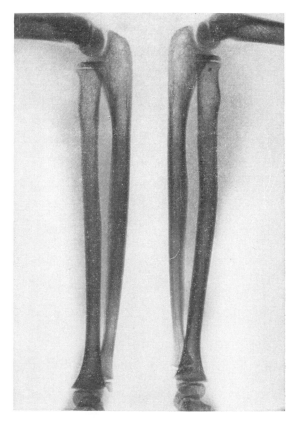

FIG. 138. L. B., 11/8/40, lateral view of the preceding case. The forearms were symmetrical. Clinically they cannot be distinguished. [Reproduced with permission of the Journal of the Ameri-Medical Association (52).]

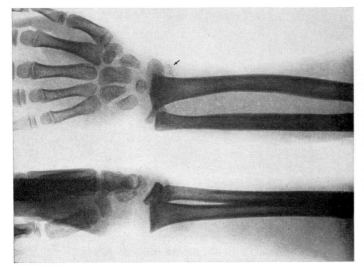

FIG. 139. R. E., male, age 10, 8/18/39. Epiphyseal fracture of the distal end of both bones of the right forearm caused by a fall from a straw stack. Note the chip of metaphysis attached to the radial epiphyseal fragment (arrow). Reduction was easy under general anesthesia. A long cast was applied for three weeks.

FIG. 140. R. E., 9/11/39. Roentgenogram of the preceding epiphyseal fracture on removal of the cast. Examination ten weeks later showed normal function.

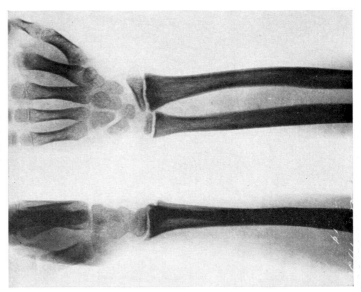

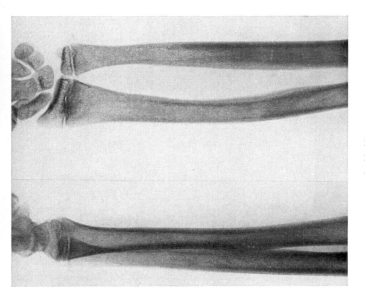

Fig. 141. R. E., 10/28/44. A five year followup showed normal function with 5 mm. of shortening of the right radius.

Fig. 142. D. B., male, age 7, 3/19/37. Minimal displacement of the left distal radial epiphysis associated with a greenstick fracture of the ulna was caused by a fall on the left hand. Quite properly a cast was applied without further reduction.

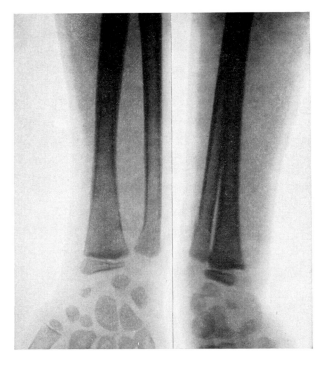

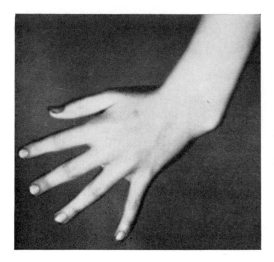

Fig. 143. D. B., 8/7/42. The injury must have been severe, with considerable damage to the growing cells of the left distal radial epiphysis because this deformity appeared in the succeeding five years.

Fig. 144. D. B., 8/7/42. An anteroposterior roentgenogram of both wrists showing marked retardation of growth at the left distal radial epiphysis.

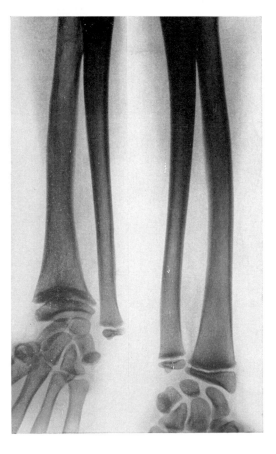

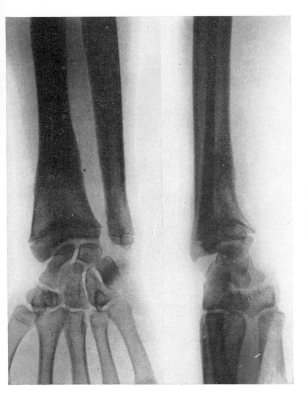

Fig. 145. D. B., 8/3/43. One year after arrest of growth of the distal ulnar epiphysis and osteotomy with insertion of a bone block in the radius. The operation on the radius stimulated further growth at both ends of the bone.

Fig. 146. D. B., 7/11/50. A good cosmetic result. Shortening of a forearm is not of great consequence. The deformity could not have been prevented but could have been corrected earlier with less sacrifice of length.

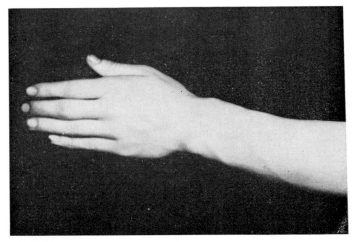

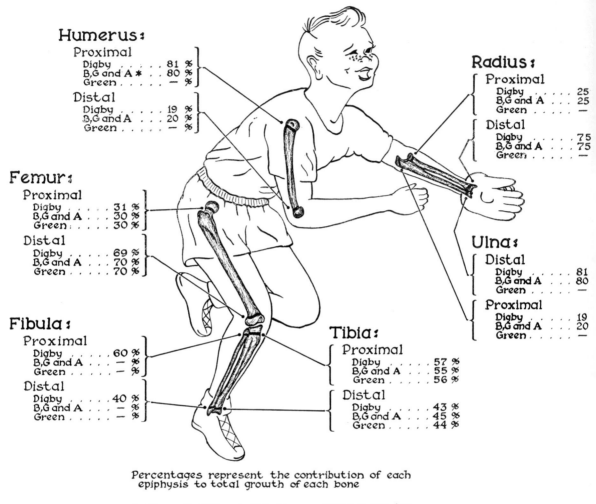

Humerus:
Proximal
Digby . . . . . 81 %
B,G and A * . . 80 %
Green . . . . . — %
Distal
Digby . . . . . 19 %
B,G and A . . . 20 %
Green . . . . . — %

Femur:
Proximal
Digby . . . . . 31 %
B,G and A . . . 30 %
Green . . . . . 30 %
Distal
Digby . . . . . 69 %
B,G and A . . . 70 %
Green . . . . . 70 %

Fibula:
Proximal
Digby . . . . . 60 %
B,G and A . . . — %
Green . . . . . — %
Distal
Digby . . . . . 40 %
B,G and A . . . — %
Green . . . . . — %

Radius:
Proximal
Digby 25
B,G and A . . . 25
Green . . . . . —
Distal
Digby 75
B,G and A . . . 75
Green . . . . . —

Ulna:
Distal
Digby 81
B,G and A . . . 80
Green . . . . . —
Proximal
Digby 19
B,G and A . . . 20
Green . . . . . —

Tibia:
Proximal
Digby . . . . . 57 %
B,G and A . . . 55 %
Green . . . . . 56 %
Distal
Digby . . . . . 43 %
B,G and A . . . 45 %
Green . . . . . 44 %

Percentages represent the contribution of each
epiphysis to total growth of each bone

*-Bisgard, Gill and Abbott.   K. Heiple, M.D. '53.

Fig. 147. Epiphyseal contributions to longitudinal bone growth. In making a prognosis as to growth stimulation or retardation resulting from epiphyseal injury, one must consider the relative normal rate of growth of the epiphysis involved. The averages are well shown in the above cartoon. (Courtesy of Dr. Charles Frantz.)

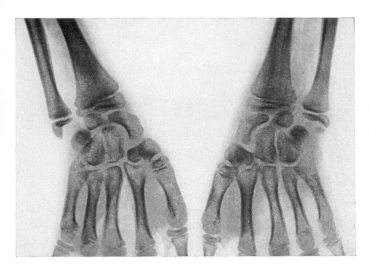

Fig. 148. A. P. L., female, age 8. This was not a fracture of the distal radial epiphysis on both sides. It was Madelung's deformity, idiopathic shortening and bowing of the radius. (Courtesy of Dr. W. W. Hurst.)

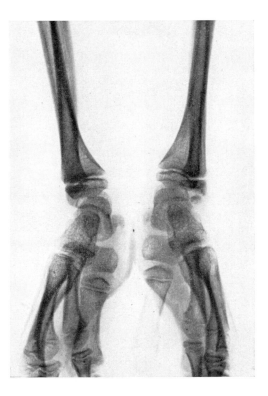

Fig. 148. B. P. L. Lateral views of the wrists of the preceding case to show the unusual volar deviation of the distal end of the radius with increase in the normal radial articular angle. (Courtesy of Dr. W. W. Hurst.)

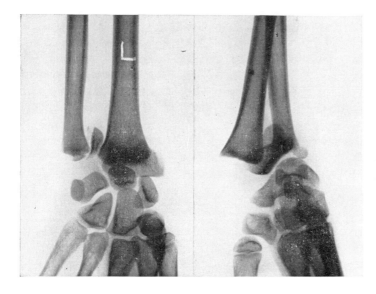

Fig. 149. E. L., male, 5/23/53. Complete dislocation of the distal epiphyses of the left forearm with fracture of the ulnar styloid when a tractor overturned with the boy's arm caught in the steering wheel. (Courtesy of Dr. Robert House.)

Fig. 150. E. L., 5/29/53 A. Reduction of the radial epiphysis was easily accomplished. The ulnar epiphysis remained caught in the distal radial articulation. It could be dislodged only with an open reduction. B shows accurate replacement of the ulnar epiphysis with pin fixation. (Courtesy of Dr. Robert House.)

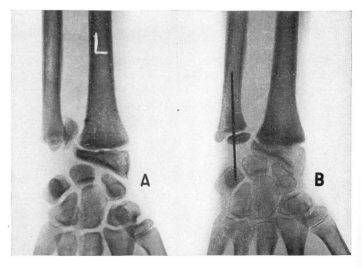

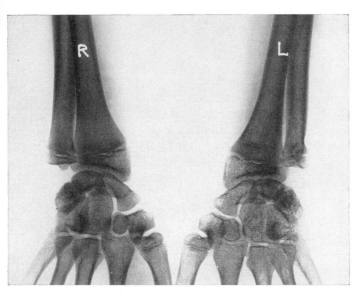

FIG. 151. E. L., 5/28/54 (at 6′ distance), one year after the preceding roentgenograms. There has been slight retardation of growth of the left radius (closed reduction) but considerably less growth of the left ulna (open reduction of the epiphysis).

Right radius......22.7 cm.
Left radius.......21.8 cm.
_____
.9 cm.

Right ulna.......25.3 cm.
Left ulna........24.0 cm.
_____
1.3 cm.

Function was good. (Courtesy of Dr. Robert House.)

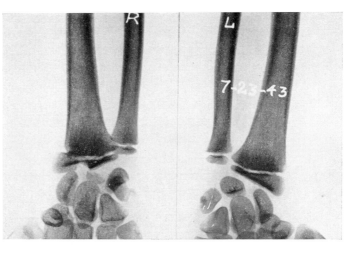

FIG. 152. G. B., male, age 12, 7/23/43. A crushing type of epiphyseal fracture of the right distal radial epiphysis with a fracture dislocation of the semilunar. Closed manipulation accurately reduced the radial epiphysis but was ineffectual in restoring the semilunar.

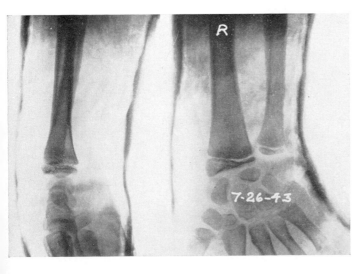

FIG. 153. G. B., 7/26/43, the wrist shown in Figure 152. On 7/24/43 the semilunar was reduced by open operation through a volar incision and a cast applied. No internal fixation was necessary.

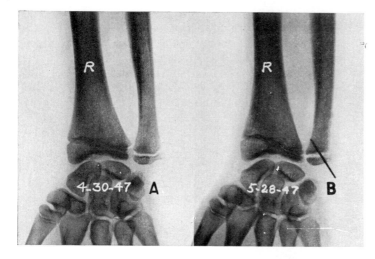

FIG. 154. G. B., 4/30/47. A shows maintenance of good position of the semilunar with retardation of growth of the radius. 5/28/47. B. The distal ulnar epiphysis had been curetted, packed with bone chips and pinned.

FIG. 155. G. B., 1/11/50. 3.6 cm shortening of the right radius was not a great handicap. Function was normal.

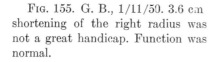

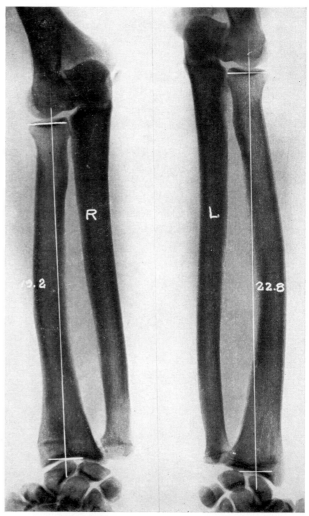

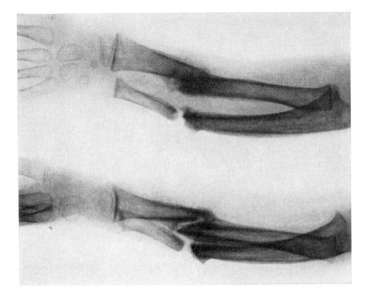

FIG. 156. D. R., male, age 5, 1/29/38. Ununited pathologic fracture of both bones of the left forearm six months following a wringer injury with slough of the skin. The fracture occurred forty days before this roentgenogram. Resection of the radius and debridement of the ulna shortened the forearm. There was spontaneous healing of the radius in eight weeks.

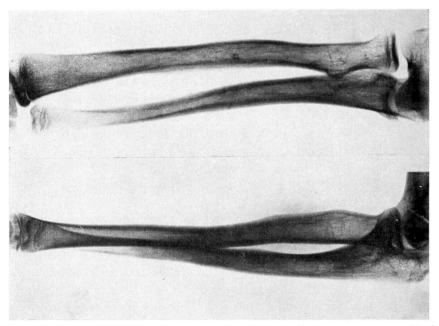

FIG. 157. D. R., 4/30/50, twelve years after the preceding roentgenogram. At eight months the left ulna was still ununited. After six years, both bones were solidly united. At twelve years, pronation was limited 10°, ulnar adduction limited 40°, volar flexion limited 10°. Other wrist motions were normal. Grip normal. The left radius was 2.9 cm. short; the left ulna, 4.2 cm. as compared to the bones of the right side in a six foot plate.

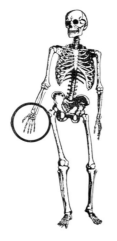

CHAPTER VI

Injuries of the Hand[3]

The child's most frequent injury is to his hand. Wide recuperative and corrective healing powers aid the surgeon but do not free him from the obligation of intelligent management. One who treats hand fractures must be prepared to treat all injured structures concomitantly. Much of the child's future social activity and economic position is dependent on the preservation of good hand function.

Sprains and dislocations are relatively common among the closed injuries to the hand. Fractures are more often open than closed, and accompanied by serious soft tissue injuries. Most statistical analyses of children's fractures have a low hand incidence—7 per cent to 10 per cent. This undoubtedly results from the omission of the most frequent hand fracture of all—the distal phalanx in the crushed finger tip. Treatment of this injury at the office or out-patient level excludes it from tabulation in a hospital series.

Most closed injuries occur with falls, playground or athletic accidents. Open injuries come from crushes in doors, and injuries by toys. Care of open and closed types is so different that they will be considered separately.

CLOSED FRACTURES AND DISLOCATIONS

The treatment of the closed fracture and dislocation has for its goals prevention of further displacement and added damage to soft parts, reduction to positions of normal bony architectural relations, and retention of the correct alignment during healing (61). Though early reduction is essential, no manipulation should be done until the exact diagnosis is established

[3] This chapter was contributed by Dr. William H. Frackelton, Assistant Professor of Surgery, Marquette University, School of Medicine.

and skilled attention can be supplied. Meanwhile, splinting of the hand and forearm in position of function (Fig. 158) with a sterile compression dressing satisfies the first-aid requirements (Fig. 159).

Diagnosis. Inspect for swelling, ecchymosis, deformity, and loss of function. Gentle palpation may reveal bony irregularities. If the child is old enough to cooperate, points of tenderness and referred pain can be located, especially in phalanges and metacarpals. Gentle compression of a digit against its proximal joint may direct attention to fracture or ligament-joint instability.

Roentgenograms are obligatory for diagnosis, record, and followup. Volar dorsal and lateral views are more satisfactorily obtained when the small child's hand is stabilized against the cassette by an overlying radiotranslucent sheet of aluminum or glass. This simple procedure prevents movement or the superimposition of curled phalanges. Symmetrical films of the opposite hand are of great aid in differentiating fracture-dislocations from the normal translucent zones at the growth centers.

Reduction is accomplished early with greater ease and with less damage to surrounding parts than under a delayed treatment program. Manipulative reduction requires satisfactory relaxation. Often local anesthesia will suffice. A preliminary barbiturate sedative and infiltration of the fracture hematoma or joint space of a dislocation with 2 per cent procaine is satisfactory for children from three years upward.

Gentleness is essential. Force leads to contusion, edema, and circulatory impairment. If reduction is not readily obtained by closed methods, attempts should not be continued. Operative reduction may be indicated. Specifically, closed reduction is likely to be ineffectual in dislocation of the metacarpophalangeal joint of the thumb, because the head of the metacarpal protrudes through the capsular rupture and between the tendinous ends of the flexor pollicis brevis where it is imprisoned. Less frequently this is true for fracture or dislocation of the head of a phalanx or of the head of a metacarpal into its joint.

Most fractures and dislocations are correctly treated in simple fashion. Too often "over treatment" leads to complications. Merely placing the hand in position of function (Fig. 158) will accomplish reduction and the proper position for retention splinting in almost all phalangeal and metacarpal fractures of the hand. The exceptions are the three "B's": Bennett's, Boxer's, and Baseball type fractures. The dorsal "bowing" of metacarpal and midphalangeal fractures is corrected with the relaxation of the wrist extensors, the long finger flexors, and the interossei. This is accomplished when the hand is in the position of function. An angular deformity of a phalanx with the apex in the ulnar or radial direction will persist for many months in a small child and will be permanent in an older

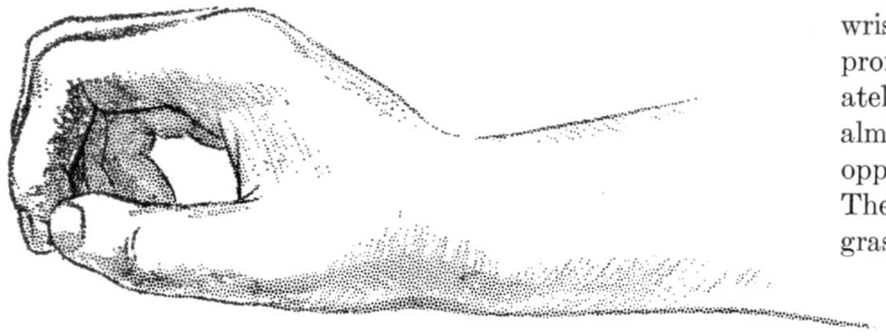

Hand in the
"Position of function"

FIG. 158. "Position of Function" wrist dorsiextended 20° to 30°, proximal and distal joints moderately flexed and midjoints flexed almost to right angles, thumb in opposition, away from the palm. The whole hand is in a "ready to grasp" position.

one. There is considerable leeway when the angular deformity has the apex in the direction of flexion, that is with the fragments hyperextended at the time of healing (Figs. 160, 161). Somewhat less correction takes place when a phalanx heals in an angulated position with the apex dorsally (Chapter I).

In obtaining or maintaining reduction of oblique, comminuted, or joint fractures, traction may be helpful. This is adequately and practically obtained by applying gauze strips held to the digit with collodion. This simple method is sufficiently secure for the application of traction necessary for phalangeal and metacarpal fracture control. A specific technic is necessary to avoid constriction. One inch wide gauze bandage is used. A length slightly over twice that of the finger is cut. With the finger in extension, the skin of the lateral sides is painted with collodion. The gauze is applied in loop fashion, the free ends of the gauze at the lateral sides of the base of the finger, and the loop extended beyond the tip of the finger. Additional collodion is painted on in successive layers as it drys. Since there is a strip of exposed skin both dorsally and volarly, circumferential constriction is avoided. The collodion is allowed to dry well before actual traction is applied to the loop (Fig. 162).

Pulp traction through a transfixion wire is unnecessary and too frequently complicated by soft tissue damage from infection or impaired circulation. Traction by means of a hole in the finger nail is unsatisfactory and damaging to the nail. Woven constricting devices such as "Japanese finger traps" are unthinkable. Adhesive tape applied in spiral fashion is likewise dangerous.

Since the amount of traction necessary rarely exceeds the capabilities of the collodion strip method, skeletal traction is seldom necessary. A thin Kirschner wire or metal traction pin may be placed through the bone transversely at the distal end of a fractured bone, or in the terminal phalanx of the finger. The hand and injured finger or fingers should be supported in a position of function on a volar curved metal splint integrated into a hand-forearm cast. Multiple digit injuries may be better supported upon a hand-forearm "position of function" splint (Fig. 159).

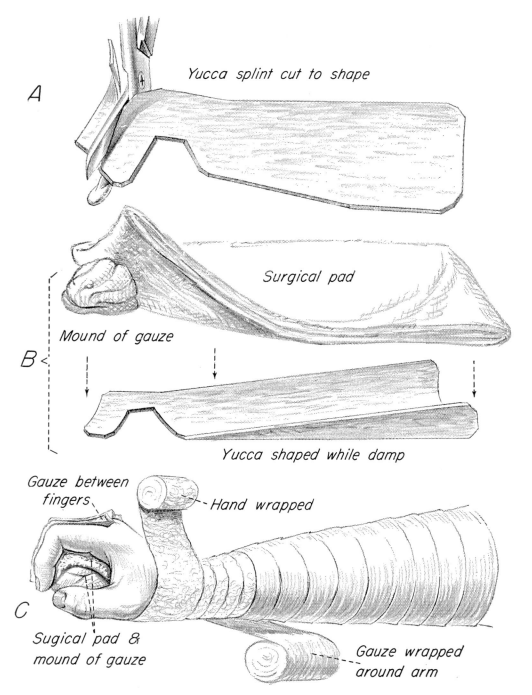

Yucca splint cut to shape

A

B

Mound of gauze

Surgical pad

Yucca shaped while damp

Gauze between fingers

Hand wrapped

C

Sugical pad & mound of gauze

Gauze wrapped around arm

FIG. 159. Hand-forearm splint and dressing. A. Yucca board soaked with water is easily cut and bent to proper shape. B. A mound of gauze gives proper palmar arch. A surgical pad over this gauze and the splint aids in protection and compression. C. Gauze is placed between the fingers; Kerlix about the hand, before applying the exterior layer of gauze bandage.

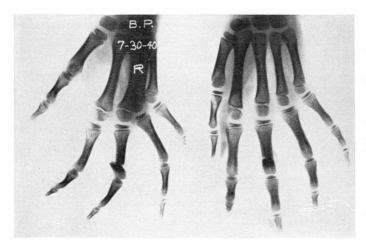

Fig. 160. B. P., female, age 8, 7/30/40. Two weeks before this roentgenogram was taken the patient sustained a fracture of the basal phalanx of the middle finger when she was struck by a flying handle. The finger had been splinted in flexion with the present deformity. Union had occurred and the deformity was allowed to remain. Symmetrical roentgenograms were taken but the left one was omitted to save space.

Fig. 161. B. P., 3/11/53. Roentgenograms thirteen years following the fracture in Figure 160 shows complete restoration of the fractured bone. The range of motion of the adjacent joints was clinically normal and symmetrical with that of the other hand. Moral: Angulation of a fracture in the plane of motion of a hinge joint disappears to a remarkable degree, particularly if the apex is toward the flexor side (Chapter I).

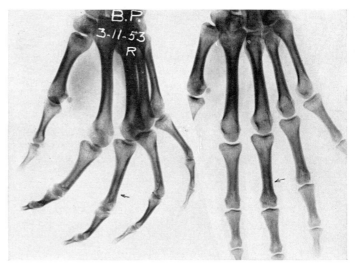

Exceptions to Reduction in the Position of Function

The three "B's" are reduced in different fashion although by closed methods. *Bennett's fracture* of the base of the thumb metacarpal through the joint and with dislocation of the "hook", is not seen in young children. When it occurs in adolescents, skeletal fixation through the head or shaft of the proximal phalanx of the thumb is the treatment.

Boxer's fracture of the neck of the metacarpal, is reduced by right angle flexion of the proximal phalanx on the metacarpal. The head of the metacarpal is stabilized in position by its joint ligaments. The usual method of applying a posterior plaster slab to hand and forearm continued

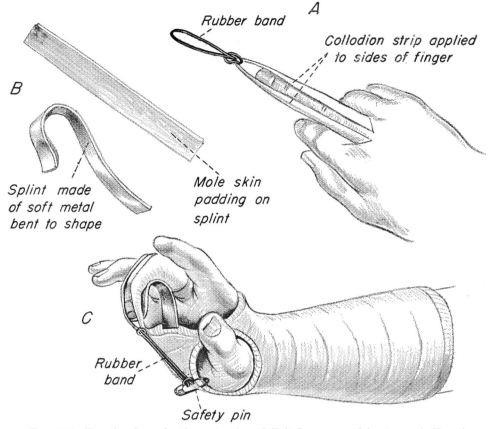

FIG. 162. Traction for reduction-retention of digital metacarpal fractures. A. Traction
is obtained by securing gauze strips to the lateral aspects of the finger by painting the
finger with a few layers of collodion. B. The commercial aluminum splint can be bent to
shape or a strip of metal fashioned to a similar design. C. A hand-forearm cast is applied
and allowed to set. The metal splint is then incorporated with additional turns of plaster.
Moleskin or gauze separates the finger from direct contact with the metal splint. When the
plaster and the collodion are sufficiently dry, correc traction car be applied by a rubber
band.

on over the proximal phalanx in its right angle position may at times be
ineffective for continued fixation.

It is suitable in older children to pass a Kirschner wire through the
head of the metacarpal on into the shaft of the metacarpal to emerge
dorsally and slightly obliquely to the long axis of the shaft and on out
through the skin proximally. Excess Kirschner wire is cut off distally.
The proximal end of the Kirschner wire emerging on the dorsum of the
hand is then pulled further proximally until the distal end of the Kirschner
wire is withdrawn beyond the metacarpal joint surface and entirely within
the head of the metacarpal. The protruding end is cut off, bent, and buried

under the skin. A metal strip splint padded with moleskin and bent at right angles can be applied on the dorsum of the hand and beyond its right angle bend to the dorsum of the proximal phalanx. Such a splint may be removed intermittently during the third to fifth week of the healing time for skin care and general cleansing.

Baseball fracture, or mallet finger, is rupture of the extensor tendon and/or fracture of the dorsum of the base of the distal phalanx. This injury is fairly frequent in children; often in an open wound. It is reduced and maintained with the distal joint in hyperextension and the midjoint of the digit in flexion, thereby securing the greatest relaxation to the extensor tendon apparatus at the distal joint. It is splinted in this position rather than by operative fixation, even if it is an open injury.

A plaster of Paris splint is often advocated but is difficult to apply and maintain in children. Satisfactory fixation is obtained by a narrow metal gutter splint padded with moleskin and placed volarly. The splint is so bent as to allow for hyperextension at the distal joint, right angle flexion at the midjoint, slight flexion at the proximal joint, and with sufficient splint length to extend proximally within the palm. It is held in place by strips of adehsive applied about the palm, the proximal phalanx, the midphalanx, and over a small felt pad placed on the dorsum of the distal joint. Weekly or biweekly adjustments are necessary during the succeeding five to six week healing period.

Open Reduction

A closed fracture of the hand of a child is operated upon only when manipulation fails to produce a satisfactory result. A well equipped operating room; good lighting; adequate assistance and instruments; complete anesthesia, usually general; and a bloodless field obtained by the use of a pneumatic cuff about the upper arm; careful skin preparation and draping are essential.

Of closed fractures and dislocations requiring open reduction, the most common is dislocation of the metacarpophalangeal joint of the thumb. We have discussed the reasons why closed reduction is likely to fail. If hyperextension of the proximal phalanx and gentle rocking to free the metacarpal head has been ineffective, a radiolateral incision is made over the proximal joint. The skin and subjacent tissue are elevated. The digital nerve is visualized and protected. The volar capsule rent is enlarged longitudinally to expose the protruding metacarpal head. The encircling tendinous portions of the flexor pollicis brevis are withdrawn from each side of the metacarpal head and reduction then obtained by manipulation under direct vision. The joint is fixed in moderate flexion for three weeks and then motion is allowed. Some limitation in range is to be expected. The longer the period before reduction, the greater will be the ultimate restriction of motion.

Metacarpophalangeal dislocations of the fingers develop a somewhat similar obstacle to closed reduction, but less frequently. The proximal joint of the index or little finger can be approached from the radial or ulnar lateral side respectively. For the middle and ring finger a dorsal incision splitting the extensor tendon and dorsal joint capsule allows direct entrance into the joint. A blunt tipped probe of dissecting type gently frees the volar capsule from the metacarpal head and permits reduction.

Interphalangeal joint fractures of the chip type or dislocations may require open exposure. This is done on the lateral side of involvement. Interposed capsular ligament is withdrawn out of the joint and reduction secured. If simple flexion position does not readily maintain correct alignment of a phalangeal head fracture, pinning of the head on the shaft with an oblique fine wire may be required. Maintenance of reduction is secured by immobilization of the bony injury area. It is secured with apparatus or bandaging that prevents motion at site of injury. This apparatus or bandaging should not interfere with circulation by constriction or pressure.

Except as previously discussed for the three "B" fractures, position of function is indicated during retention. Normal concavity of the palm preserves the arch of the hand. The wrist is in 30° dorsiextension, the metacarpophalangeal and distal interphalangeal joints in 45° of flexion, and the middle interphalangeal joint in almost 90° of flexion. For multiple digit injury a position of function metal splint of the Mason-Allen type is ideal although not commercially available in a child's size. An unpadded splint made from plaster strips is highly satisfactory. For multiple digit injury, the plaster splint can extend distally and volarly sufficient to form the flexion support for the digits. Unless the thumb is involved it is advantageously left free of plaster even to its base For one or two digits the plaster need not extend farther than the distal palmar crease. The involved digits can be supported on a volar curved metal splint integrated into the plaster. Freeing the uninvolved digits for movement is practical though not so essential in children as in adults. The tendency for stiffening of uninvolved but splinted fingers is less in the child than in the adult.

If traction with the collodion gauze loop is to be used, a rubber band from the loop is fastened with a safety pin into the plaster cast at the navicular volar wrist area (Fig 162).

Small children have an amazing ability to remove dressings and splints. The only satisfactory counter move is to fix the entire limb from finger tips to the upper arm in a complete cast, or a plaster splint for part of the circumference of the arm. The latter is applied over light padding with

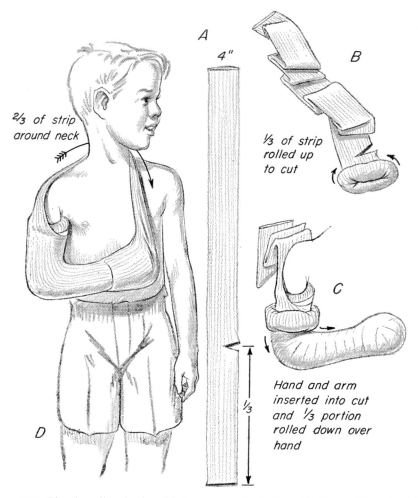

FIG. 163. Fixation sling for hand injury cases. A. A 3″ or 4″ (7 cm.–10 cm.) width of stockinet is cut to proper length and notched as shown. B. The short third is rolled back. C. The notched opening and the roll of stockinet are passed over the hand and splint dressing to an upper arm position. The short third is then unrolled to cover the forearm and hand. D. The remaining length is passed about the shoulder and neck and slipped over the hand. The end is secured with safety pins with the hand at the proper height. The safety pins are covered with adhesive tape.

the elbow at right angles and maintained in place with a spiral gauze bandage. In addition, a halter type of stockinet sling (Fig. 163) will add comfort as well as prevent the destruction or dislodging of the cast through the child's banging, dunking, or other activities.

The use of Kirschner wires at time of reduction has been mentioned. Occasionally they may also be used transversely for metacarpal fractures, especially oblique ones. Even here position of function splinting and gentle collodion strip gauze traction will ordinarily suffice. Wiring or plating of hand fractures is unnecessary in children.

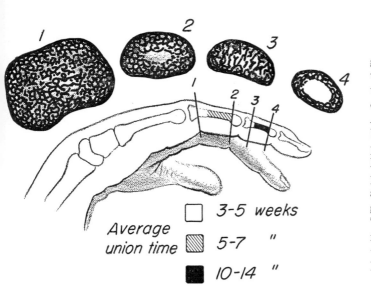

FIG. 164. The level of a phalangeal fracture affects the healing time. At the base of the phalanx, the bone is more vascular and cancellous. Healing is more rapid. At midshaft, the amount of cortical bone is greatest and vascularity proportionately less; healing time here is slowest. At the head of the phalanx, cancellous bone is not as abundant as at the base but is in greater proportion than in midshaft. The figures given may be decreased for children down to one-half for toddlers. [Redrawn from Dr. Eric Moberg (58).]

In the early post injury stage, elevation is desirable. It is mandatory in the severely contused limb. When the patient is in bed, the upper arm is horizontal and the forearm at right angles and vertical to it. The arm is suspended by a loop of bandage passed along either side of the forearm and underneath the elbow. In the ambulatory patient the halter stockinet sling will prevent dependency. Immobilization should be continuous until healing of soft tissues and firm bony union have been established.

Ligamentous and capsular injuries accompanying dislocations require two weeks of complete immobilization. During the third week the hand may be removed from the splint for bathing, but should be splinted between the dressings.

The healing of fractures of the phalanges and metacarpals requires immobilization for three to five weeks in children. Distal phalangeal fractures will tolerate activity somewhat earlier. Phalangeal fractures vary in healing time with the level at which the fracture occurs. There is hard, slow healing, cortical bone in the midshaft position. Near the head or base of a phalanx, there is more cancellous vascular bone (Fig. 164). In the mid portion of the shaft healing is slower by one to two weeks. Maintenance of reduction must be timed accordingly.

Carpal fractures rarely occur in children except with direct crushing injuries (Chapter V, Fractures of the Forearm and Wrist).

After immobilization is discontinued, the program is different for the child than for the adult. Formal occupational or physical therapy treatments are unnecessary. The restoration of function will occur through the child's own hand activity as he plays with his toys or engages in ordinary games. Indeed, attempts at passive stretching may prolong and increase disability of sprains and joint involvements. A sprained joint, with or without ligamentous tear, may require two to three months of use before maximum mobility and subsidence or thickening has come about. It will recover best without passive manipulations.

Open Fractures and Dislocations

Open hand injuries with fractures and dislocations require composite care of all damaged tissues (60). Such wounds may involve damage to skin by burning or avulsion, laceration of nerves and tendons, and open injuries of bones and joints. In so complex a "machine" as the hand in which there are over two hundred named parts, single tissue injuries are a rarity. Success in treatment depends upon simultaneous or proper sequential treatment of all injured tissues.

The initial first aid care of open hand injuries (61) is aimed at protection. Avoidance of infection, added trauma, and future disability are the goals. The application of a sterile gentle compression dressing to the hand, and splinting in position of function satisfies these requirements. Even the hemorrhage from a severed radial artery can be controlled by the gentle compression. The sterile dressing protects the open wound from contamination by interested bystanders or dirty instruments. The splint and dressing immobilize the hand and prevent added tearing, separation, or piercing of damaged tissue.

Preliminary to definitive treatment of open hand injuries, the *"how when, and where"* history should be obtained. The manner of injury—"how"—will give an index as to the type of wound and the severity of the crush factor present. An estimate of forthcoming edema and fibrosis, and the consequent limitations for operative manipulation is thus gained. If the time interval is not too great—"when"—(four to six hours) an open contaminated wound can be converted to a clean one. Primary closure is then desirable. The place—"where"—the accident occurred will give further index as to contamination—did it happen in the manured farm field, or in the relatively clean area of the household kitchen? Inquiry as to first aid treatment gives further information as to possible added contamination and trauma.

Diagnosis prior to the child's entrance into an operating room is limited to functional testing rather than examination of the wound itself. Can the patient flex the distal joint of the finger against resistance? If not, likely the profundus tendon is cut. Can the patient perceive the touch of a cotton applicator to the digit surface? If not, perhaps the digital nerve to that area has been severed or severely contused. Can the patient extend the last two joints of his fingers, spread his fingers apart, and bring them together? If not, likely the motor ulnar nerve has been damaged. Can the patient bring the thumb out as in the position of reaching for a glass? If not, there is probably damage to the median motor nerve. All of these tests can be carried out without removing the gauze covering the wound. If the child is too young for cooperation or understanding, functional testing is of little worth. Inspection as to deformity and the location of the wound will have to serve as a guide to probable damage.

Roentgenograms are taken without disturbing the overlying dressing. Under operating room conditions, with masked nose and mouth, an adequate wound examination can be made by sterile handling.

Definitive treatment. The patient is treated systematically for pain, shock, and hemorrhage and surveyed for other injuries which may require concomitant or priority care. Antibiotics are given prophylactically. Tetanus toxoid booster (tetanus antitoxin in the absence of prior active immunization) is administered (Chapter XVI).

For *operative treatment*, the following are essential: a well equipped operating room, good lighting, adequate assistance and instruments, complete anesthesia (almost invariably general), and a bloodless field secured by small pneumatic cuff to the upper arm. The area about the wound is gently and thoroughly cleansed with white soap or bland detergent and water. Saline irrigation of the wound along with instrumental removal of devitalized tissue and foreign bodies completes the mechanical cleansing.

When the crush or contamination factor is significant, or the wound is many hours old, repair and closure are deferred. Nonetheless, mechanical cleansing is carried out gently, but thoroughly. The highest goal of immediate definitive care of hand injury is healing without infection. Friedrich (68) said in essence, most wounds contaminated with certain pathogenic bacteria, but cleansed by mechanical flushing within six hours will heal without infection. Most wounds contaminated similarly but not so cleansed until after six hours will develop infection. If this six hour time interval is not exceeded, severed structures may be repaired and the wound closed primarily. When surface tissue has been lost but closure is otherwise indicated, a skin graft facilitates closure without tension and is nature's "best bandage". A voluminous gentle compression dressing is applied and the hand and forearm splinted with metal or plaster in optimum position of function. Post-operative elevation and rest of the hand promote healing.

Noninterference with the initial dressing (six to ten days) permits undisturbed healing. Early evidence of infection is elevated temperature, odor, and pain in that sequence. Gangrene is indicated by pain, odor, and temperature ("Top" and "Pot"). Active motion is started when the structures are sufficiently healed; usually ten days for skin and subjacent tissues, two to three weeks for muscle, fascia, and capsule, and three weeks

or more for tendons and nerves. Supervised passive motion may be instituted earlier in certain instances. The schedule for bone and joint healing
has been listed previously.

During operation, joint dislocations are reduced. Bone fragments in
the open wound are restored as nearly as possible to normal position. They
are almost invariably saved when any periosteum with blood supply remains attached. Even detached pieces may be put back into position
except in highly contaminated wounds. Loose bodies that could cause
joint irritation are removed.

In open fractures, reduction without foreign material fixation is best.
Occasionally it may be necessary to stabilize the fractures with a suture
of stainless steel wire or a stainless steel pin. Maintenance of reduction of
fractures or dislocations can usually be obtained by appropriate splinting
in position of function. If traction is required and contusion of the skin of
the fingers makes collodion strip application unwise, then a transverse
pin may be inserted in the distal phalanx.

Tendons are seldom repaired when a fracture exists in the same wound
area (63). Only fine nonabsorbable suture such as 00000, or 0000 silk or
nylon, or fine stainless steel wire (No. 35 or 36, .0056 or .005 inch; .013 or
.0125 cm.) are used. Crushed, severed ends of tendons are minimally debrided to maintain length. Maintenance of approximation depends not on
strength of suture, but on relaxation by splinting. Tendons are relatively
avascular and particularly susceptible to infection and indurated healing.
Additional operative trauma may be disastrous. Suture by intratendinous
crisscross suture using a double arm twelve inch strand is a suitable technic (Fig. 165). Suture is passed transversely through the tendon ⅜" (9
mm.) or so from the proximal cut end. The needles pass alternately transversely and somewhat obliquely to emerge at the end of the tendon. They
are similarly inserted and crisscrossed in the distal end of the tendon
emerging ultimately on the same side at an area near to each other and
again about ⅜" (9 mm.) away from the severed end. Each end of the
strand is pulled individually and alternately to tighten and "accordio-
nate" the tendon into firm approximation before tying the suture. The
suture is placed transversely in a single plane. By this technic there is
minimal aseptic necrosis from the presence of the suture and no circumferential strangulation.

In the narrow channel of the tendon sheath within the finger, adherence
of the injured flexor tendon is all too common. "No man's land" lies between the distal crease of the palm and the midflexion crease of the finger.
Primary tendon suture seldom succeeds here even when the sublimis tendon is removed; it invariably fails when both tendons are united within
the sheath. It is invariably unsuccessful when a fracture coexists at the

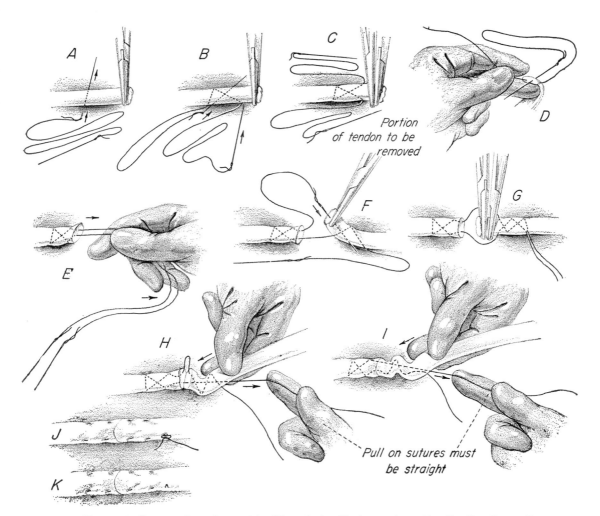

FIG. 165. Suture of tendons with silk technic. [Redrawn from Dr. Sterling Bunnell (59).] A· to D. With a thread and two needles the sutures are placed traversing the tendon with each needle from two to four times and emerging through the end. E. All slack is drawn out. F. and G. The suture is continued similarly up the other tendon. Both ends are brought out at the same spot. In placing the last strand in the second tendon end the needle must not spear the other thread or the threads will not slip. By keeping the needles on separate sides of the tendon this is avoided, or better, both needles may be thrust through the tendon simultaneously. H. and I. To prevent the tendon ends from separating under strain the slack is removed from the second tendon. To do this one suture is pulled at a time as the tendon is shoved along it to snug against the other tendon end. J. and K. There is but one knot; when tied it sinks into the tendon and at a place where it receives the least strain as knots are the weakest parts of a tendon suture.

same level as the tendon injury. The callus about the fracture is accompanied by induration and fixation of the tendon.

Good results accrue from secondary tendon repair after the induration of injury has subsided (three to five weeks). It is far better to gain primary wound healing in the hand and accomplish secondary flexor tendon repair than to jeopardize eventual function through complicated indurated healing. Flexor tendons distal and proximal to "no man's land" give good results when repaired within four to eight hours following a lacerated wound without a crush factor. Crush is thus another contraindication to tendon repair under almost any circumstance. Only when the contused area is so small that it can be excised, is repair feasible. Then one deals with an "incised", not a "crush" wound.

Extensor tendons are anatomically different from flexors. Although they are relatively avascular and tend to become adherent at levels of bone injury, they are not located in tubular sheaths. Simple mattress tendon suture is used. The results from extensor tendon repair are usually good.

Even after the so-called "safe time interval" for tendon repairs has passed, it is wise to unite severed nerve ends. When crush is not a factor, primary definitive neurorrhaphy can be done, 000000 eye silk suture with an atraumatic needle is used for the interrupted sutures placed in the neurilemma sheath. In crushed or grossly contaminated wounds, only temporary initial union should be sought. Secondary repair (neuroplasty with lysis of nerve, removal of neuroma and neurorrhaphy) is done later, following subsidence of induration.

Open wounds with avulsion of tissue and exposure of bone or joint, are not suitable for split thickness skin grafting. It is better to swing a pedicle of skin and subjacent tissue over to the wound from a neighboring digit or implant the wound into a subpectoral area of the trunk. The bed from which the pedicle was advanced is covered with a split thickness skin graft.

Discussion of *the crushed fingertip* merits special consideration because of its frequency (64). In a child, and especially the infant, one might hesitate to consider hospitalization and operation under general anesthesia for so small an injury. The following plan offers an adequate substitute.

If the tip is crushed but the bone is not denuded by avulsion of the soft parts, general anesthesia is unnecessary. One may use a barbiturate sedative by mouth, or for the infant by rectum; codeine by mouth or hypodermically. The fingertip is gently but thoroughly irrigated with sterile water and saline solution. Even tissue of questionable vitality is worth preserving. Approximation of the tissue is obtained by a simple collodion dressing. Narrow strips of fine mesh gauze moistened in collodion and brought over the tip of the finger in crisscross fashion will serve (Fig. 166).

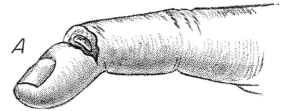

A

Overlapping collodion strips

B

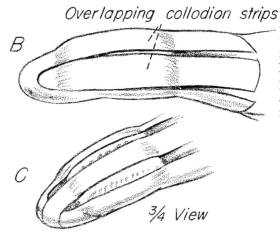

C

¾ View

FIG. 166. Treatment of crushed finger tip without suture. A. A child's crushed and lacerated finger is thoroughly cleansed. B. and C. Reduction and closure obtained by painting the finger with collodion and applying ¼″ (6 mm.) strips of fine mesh gauze.

A gently compressing dressing and splint are necessary. Tetanus immunization should be given (Chapter XVI, Open Fractures).

Fractures of the distal phalanx require no additional treatment. If the nail has been partially avulsed, it is best to trim it off proximally, to such a level that it does not overlap the epinychium. This preserves the distal end of the nail for its splinting and protective effect and yet allows exudation of hemorrhage outward from the pulp. This treatment of the nail overcomes dislocation of the soft tissue, allows reduction and alignment of comminuted portions of the distal phalanx, and serves better to counteract subsequent nail deformity.

Traumatic amputation. When an open fracture includes the loss of a part of a hand, portions of digits that are partially attached but of questionable vitality should not be amputated. The regenerative powers of the child are remarkable. The time required for healing such a digit is not important in a child. In the adult such a prolonged treatment period would be accompanied by post injury fibrosis in the other fingers. This is not true in the child.

When the amputation has been entirely completed by the injury, treatment is aimed at coverage. Further bone should not be rongeured away merely to provide a local pedicle skin flap. Instead, if local skin is insufficient, a free split thickness skin graft can be used (Fig. 167). Often it is all that is necessary for permanent recovery. If not, it will preserve the digit end for later reconstruction. When all conditions are suitable to consider the wound as converted from contaminated to clean, a denuded bony end may be covered with a cross finger pedicle skin graft from an

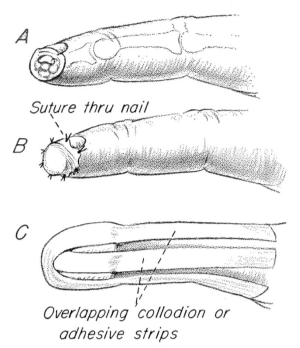

A

Suture thru nail

B

C

Overlapping collodion or
adhesive strips

FIG. 167. Free skin graft for partial amputation of finger tip. A. The length of the amputated finger tip should be preserved; the bone should not be cut back merely to obtain soft tissue closure. B. A thin "split-thickness" skin graft taken from a donor hip or forearm area is placed over the denuded tip and held with a few fine "tacking" sutures. C. A small compression pad overlying the skin graft is held in place with collodion or adhesive strips applied in crossed fashion as shown.

adjacent digit, a pedicle skin graft from the thenar eminence, or from a subpectoral pedicle. A thumb should be saved under any circumstance, for even a stiff one is very useful. A denuded thumb should be covered with a pedicle graft. A completely denuded finger, however, seldom regains satisfactory function with an encircling pedicle skin graft. Partial preservation of length, especially in a girl, may be indicated in order that a prosthesis may be applied to the stump later.

The story that the "finger was completely cut off and sewed back on as good as new" must generally be relegated to the category of old wives' tales. When the tip of a finger has been severed and that tip has not been crushed appreciably, it is feasible to use it as a composite graft, lightly stitch it in place. Treat the wound expectantly. The need for preservation of partially amputed parts or digits has already been emphasized. Survival and usefulness may be gained; failure does not constitute an added loss.

It is worthwhile to emphasize that the highest goal to be obtained in hand injury is primary healing without infection. An analysis of the wound, the appreciation of the potentialities of repair and limitation of treatment within these potentialities will best serve the patient.

The child's spontaneous hand usage is all that is needed in the way of therapy to restore form and function upon the completion of healing. Reconstructive surgery on the tissues surviving injury has wide scope. Even one surviving digit is more valuable than the most perfected mechanical hand. A single digit or a metacarpal stump can grasp or pinch against a prosthetic post attached to a glove or a forearm cuff. When the hand is totally lost, a prosthesis and early training are worthwhile.

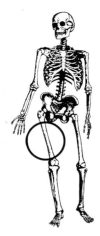

CHAPTER VII

Injuries of the Femur

THE SHAFT OF THE FEMUR

Etiology

About 70 per cent of all fractures of the shaft of the femur in children occur in the middle third, 18 per cent in the proximal third, and the remaining 12 per cent at the distal end. The distribution varies with the age.

A transverse fracture of the middle third of a child's femur (Fig. 168) is usually produced by direct trauma; a long spiral (Fig. 169), by torsion. Comminuted fractures are less common than in adults. Greenstick fractures are less frequent at this level than in the distal third. To the simple ones that occur in childhood games are added the complex injuries of the modern machine age.

Birth fractures of the femur are usually transverse of the middle third. Rarely are they complicated by a palsy of the lumbosacral plexus analogous to, but obviously much more difficult to produce than a similar lesion in the brachial plexus. This exceedingly rare nerve lesion may occur without bone injury. In making the diagnosis, one should not overlook an epiphyseal fracture.

Treatment

Closed fractures of the shaft may be treated by conservative measures with a routinely satisfactory outcome. An incomplete fracture without deformity is immobilized in a cast for six to eight weeks depending upon the age of the child. In treating the displaced fracture, only a few principles need be observed. Rotation and angulation of the distal fragment must be avoided. Both can be eliminated by traction with the legs held in symmetrical positions. In the young child this is carried out with a double overhead system (69). It is better not to tie the ropes to a rigid bar but to use separate weights and pulleys (Fig. 170). An efficient re-straint is imperative (70).

A child over five or six years is usually better controlled by single or double Russell traction with a weight of three to six pounds (Fig. 171). Pulleys must be kept oiled. An efficient foot piece will prevent rotation and keep the foot at a right angle. The knee sling must be soft and so placed as to avoid pressure on the peroneal nerve. A steady pull on the fractured leg will usually maintain correct alignment (71). Rotation is controlled by the foot piece with the occasional addition of adhesive traction with a lateral pull. If there is angulation, it may be corrected by application of traction to the other leg.

In fractures of the junction of the middle and upper thirds there is frequently adduction of the proximal fragment. This is overcome *not* by increasing the pull on the broken leg but by *diminishing* it and pulling harder with traction on the opposite side (Fig. 172). This tilts the pelvis distally on the opposite side, thus adducting the distal fragment on the affected side. If there is excessive adduction of the distal fragment, the legs can be widely separated to correct alignment. In spite of careful observation, the fracture of an unusually active child may develop early consolidation with angulation. The fracture may be rebroken easily under sedation or general anesthesia (Figs. 173–177). The callus will have a plastic consistency which will aid in maintaining correct alignment with further traction.

A traction frame for newborns and infants may be mounted on a board with a foam rubber pad (Fig. 178) so that the child may be cared for at home. Rubber bands replace the pulley traction. Nursing care is easy if the buttocks are held just off the pad. The child remains comfortable during transportation to the office or hospital for careful inspection at frequent intervals and for roentgenologic examinations. Rotation is controlled by keeping the feet in symmetrical positions. Twenty degrees of angulation apex posterior (loss of the anterior bow), and one centimeter of overriding are permissible.

There is less chance of complication and a higher percentage of good results with traction than with other forms of conservative treatment. Union is more prompt than with a cast and there is less likelihood of angulation. The disadvantage is the need for a hospital stay of three to six weeks depending upon the age of the child. In very young children, the fracture will be solid in as short a time as two weeks but traction should not be removed until the tenderness of the callus has disappeared.

There are *dangers associated with skin traction* in children which must be recognized (72). Tight bandages may cause circulatory embarrassment. If they are not released immediately, they will soon cause sloughs.

or worse, ischemic necrosis (Fig. 179). This is particularly true of overhead traction in infants. The well leg is more often injured in this manner than the broken one. Pain in the leg, swelling, cyanosis, or pallor of the toes require immediate removal of the bandages and inspection of the skin. Never disregard the complaint of pain. The pain from a fracture should not be sufficient to require opiates in a child.

Traction may be applied with ordinary adhesive plaster. Even better, is the use of reinforced flannelette strips glued on with Ace adherent. Allow the liquid to become almost dry before the strips are laid on smoothly, and held in place with a loosely applied elastic cotton bandage. Apply traction at once instead of waiting, as with adhesive plaster. Tincture of benzoin is less efficient in a child because it soon loses its hold. Displacement of the traction strips must be detected promptly. If the child kicks vigorously the circular turns of bandage will slip up around the heel and cause pressure sores. Frequent inspection and rewrapping when necessary will eliminate this complication.

Skeletal traction is rarely necessary in a child because alignment can be maintained by skin traction and complete restoration of length is not desirable in a displaced fracture (67, 73, 75). When gross shortening is not detected promptly, skeletal traction may be indicated. A Kirschner wire is to be preferred to a pin or tongs. It is better inserted through the crest of the tibia just distal to the proximal epiphysis than in the lower femur. With heavy traction, wires have cut through into the epiphyseal plates, and caused growth arrest of the femur (15) and the tibia (76). A wire distal to the tibial tubercle is safe.

The likelihood of infection is great when a transfixion wire is used in a child unless it is incorporated in plaster from the toes to well above the wire. The cast prevents contamination by lateral movement of the wire or by the child's manipulation and scratching.

The treatment of a displaced shaft fracture with a plaster cast requires considerable skill. The hips and knees should be flexed. The healing time is longer than with traction.

If the fracture is transverse and can be locked end to end with proper rotation, the only danger is that of angulation. Repeated roentgenograms are necessary. If angulation occurs, it can usually be corrected by wedging the cast. Beware of excessive local pressure or constriction. The involved femur that was end to end is usually too long after six months.

Spiral or oblique fractures of the femur are better treated with traction than a cast unless the soft parts maintain the position of the bone ends with only slight displacement. Then cast treatment is good because immobilization is all that is necessary.

It is usually a mistake to discontinue traction and apply a cast while the callus is soft. The fragments are likely to angulate. When the callus is no longer tender, traction may be discontinued safely. Then a cast or a caliper is superfluous. Keep the child in bed at home for an additional week and then permit partial weight bearing with crutches. As the child gains confidence he will automatically transfer weight from the crutches to the foot on the affected side. He will not overdo unless mischievous boys steal his crutches. In the absence of complications there is no reason to gild the lily with physical therapy.

For the transportation of a child with a fresh fracture of the femur, fixed traction may be applied with a Thomas splint. For an infant, the usual overhead may be mounted on a board (Fig. 178). Hoke traction is ideal (Fig. 180). It provides a constant pull on the affected leg by means of a ratchet with the opposite leg for countertraction. It is comfortable and may be left on for the duration of treatment. Complications are less likely than with ordinary cast fixation and healing is prompt.

In the usual displaced shaft fracture of the femur, end to end apposition is not only unnecessary but undesirable. In a large series of cases, the average overgrowth of fractured femurs was 1 cm. Then 1 cm. of overriding is the ideal position for union (77, 78, 79). Side to side apposition gives a more rapid and stronger union than end to end contact. With accelerated growth on the fractured side, the final leg lengths should be symmetrical. A fractured femur that is reduced so that its length is equal to the one on the opposite side, will likely be too long at the end of treatment. A long leg is just as undesirable as a short one.

If the fracture is not displaced, the periosteum will not be stripped. Growth will be accelerated little, if any. Then the existing normal length is desirable. It should be obvious that all fractures of the femur must be followed for a year or more, until one knows that the rate of growth is equal on the two sides, and that the legs are of about the same length.

The exact degree of *acceleration of growth* is unpredictable (67). As a general rule, the amount of overgrowth is proportional to the initial displacement of the bone ends and the amount of callus formed. The surest way to get excessive overgrowth is to remanipulate a fracture after callus is formed so as to produce a huge exuberant mass (Fig. 176). One inch or more of overgrowth has been observed repeatedly after such manipulation. In refracture of a malunited femur, traction should be adjusted to leave 1 inch of shortening (Figs. 181–183).

Inequality of leg length a year or more following a femoral fracture is a permanent deformity. There is no beneficent force that intercedes to produce "compensatory shortening" as has been naively stated (5). Accelerated growth is a physiologic, not a compensatory process. It is true that following a fracture in an older child, the overall development of the bone will be accelerated, so that epiphyseal closure takes place a few months prematurely. But during that few months before final closure, very little longitudinal growth occurs. At best the unaffected femur will gain in length only a few millimeters at the end of the growth period.

If the difference in length is a significant deformity the long femur should be stapled (80, 81) in time to equalize the length. Occasionally in a young child of short parents, the opposite femur may be stimulated (82, 83, 84, 85) so as to gain desirable height.

"Marked overriding" or "gross deformity" are usually given as indications for open reduction. There is no excuse for malposition if skin traction is used. In the case of a neglected fracture with such a deformity, refracture with skin or skeletal traction will suffice to obtain a normal extremity. In such a case intramedullary fixation is contraindicated. End to end apposition, plus the stimulation of refracture plus the irritation of the foreign body produce marked overgrowth. It is interesting to note that in Cole's records (86) abnormal bowing of the shaft "was seen only in the operated cases".

The plea that open reduction is necessary to remove interposed muscles is groundless in children. Most strands of muscle will pull out of the way with traction. Callus will form in and around fibers of muscle which remain interposed (Fig. 112). Defects in the callus that are visible in the roentgenogram as transluscent areas are soon completely obliterated and solid union results.

It is true that under ideal circumstances the immediate hazard from open reduction is small, but it is ever present. Plates and screws are particularly bad in children. They are prone to break with the inevitable constant movement, even in a plaster cast. The operation restores the exact length of the bone, which immediately starts to overgrow. The callus is scanty and weak, however, and must be protected for a long period of time. The plate must be removed later. This means an additional operation and further stimulation of growth.

The intramedullary nail is less likely to break in children than the bone plate. The cases that have been reported to me have shown overgrowth of the femur of variable amounts from one to three centimeters. The stimulation from the nail alone is probably not more than one to two centimeters. Further elongation would be dependent upon massive callus formation or low grade infection. Removal of a nail probably produces no further overgrowth.

The operation is unnecessary, however, and as such must be condemned. It introduces the hazard of an unnecessary anesthetic, unnecessary exposure of the bone ends, and trauma to the entire marrow cavity of the femur. There is no reason for doing it. With traction, in a growing child, there is solid healing within four to eight weeks. Nonunions do not occur except following open reductions. In an adult the healing time is much longer. Nonunions and delayed unions are common and there is a real reason for using the intramedullary nail.

After open reductions in children by competent surgeons we have seen a variety of serious complications: nonunion (Figs. 184, 185), osteomyelitis (Fig. 186), multiple refractures (Fig. 187), gross deformity (Fig. 188), and in one early case, death from septicemia (Fig. 189). This chamber of horrors merits the serious consideration of anyone who contemplates open reduction on the shaft of the femur in a child (87). One postoperative osteomyelitis in a lifetime is enough to cure a surgeon of a casual attitude toward open reduction. In the Milwaukee Children's Hospital there has been no serious complication with the use of traction.

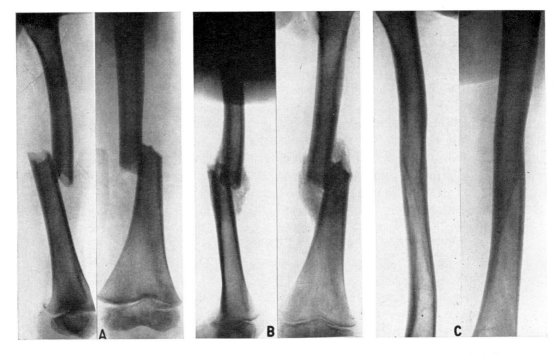

Fig. 168. K. L., male, age 4. Transverse fracture of the middle third. A. On admission. B. After three weeks of traction. Bayonet apposition with 1 cm. overriding is desirable. The angulation with the apex posteriorly could have been prevented by the support of a firm pillow. C. The same femur two years later. Molding has taken care of the bony deformity. Roentgenograms at six foot distance eight years after the fracture show that the left femur measured 7 mm. longer than the unbroken right. [Reproduced with permission of the Southern Medical Journal (87).]

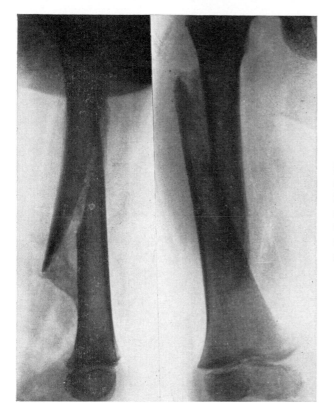

FIG. 169. H. W., male, age 4. Spiral fracture of the middle third after four weeks of traction. Union is solid with overriding and some angulation. Better position than this can usually be obtained. In eight months the length was restored and alignment corrected.

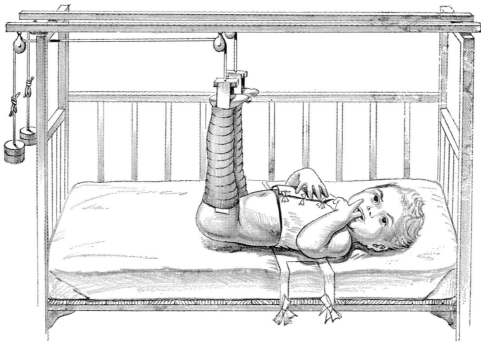

FIG. 170. Byrant originally applied vertical traction to only the fractured femur. It is better to pull on both legs. Traction may be adjusted better if separate weights and pulleys are used. Some form of restraint is imperative.

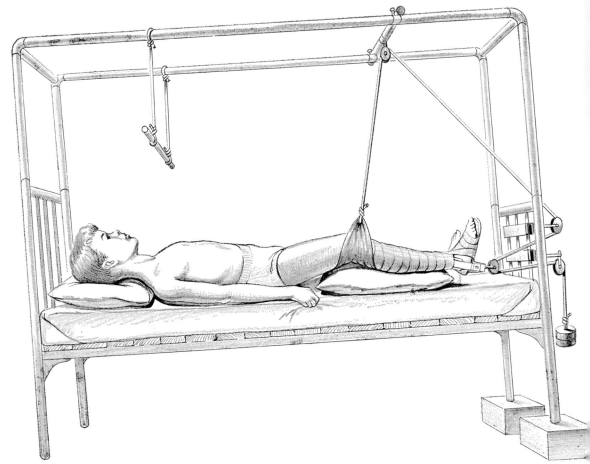

FIG. 171. Russell traction is ideal for the treatment of fracture of the femur in older
children. If the position is difficult to maintain the other leg should be treated similarly.
If the child is cooperative, unilateral traction may be used. A box is then placed at the foot
of the bed for counterpressure on the well foot as an alternative to elevation of the foot end
of the bed.

A
Incorrect

B
Correct

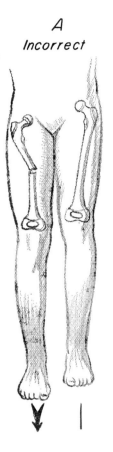
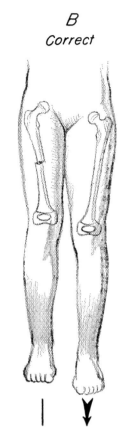

FIG. 172. When the proximal fragment is adducted (A), do not increase the pull; apply traction to the other leg (B), tilt the pelvis downward on the other side and release the adductor spasm.

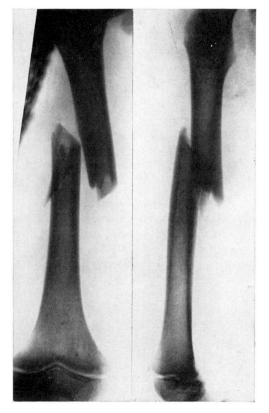

FIG. 173. G. K., male, age 6, 12/1/33. Fracture of the right femur in an automobile accident. [Reproduced with permission of the American Academy of Orthopaedic Surgeons, Instructional Course Lectures (142).]

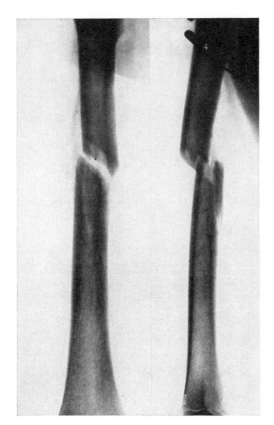

FIG. 174. G. K., 12/15/33, two weeks after the previous roentgenogram. Satisfactory apposition but with overpull. Beginning callus formation. [Reproduced with permission of the American Academy of Orthopaedic Surgeons, Instructional Course Lectures (142).]

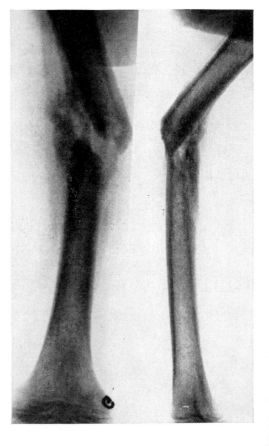

FIG. 175. G. K., 1/13/34. At six weeks the Russell traction was removed. The fragments angulated and refractured. With 1 cm. of overlap, union would have been solid.

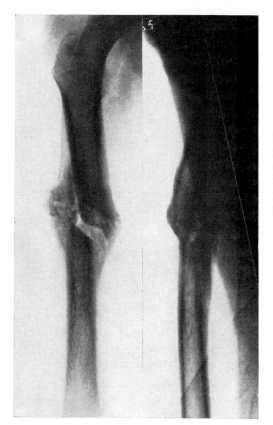

Fig. 176. G. K., 1/30/34. Three weeks after the reapplication of Russell traction, the callus was mature (not tender). There is now end to end apposition with massive callus. Overgrowth was inevitable in such a case. [Reproduced with permission of the American Academy of Orthopaedic Surgeons, Instructional Course Lectures (142).]

Fig. 177. G. K., 11/8/40, seven years after figure 176. One inch (2.5 cm.) overgrowth of the right femur has persisted. A Phemister epiphysiodesis was performed at the distal end of the right femur with satisfactory equalization of leg length. [Reproduced with permission of the American Academy of Orthopaedic Surgeons, Instructional Course Lectures (142).]

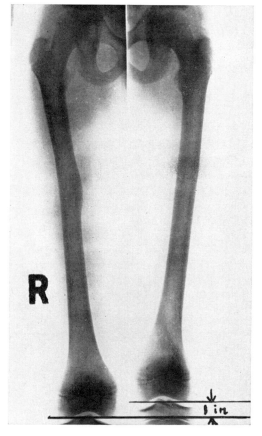

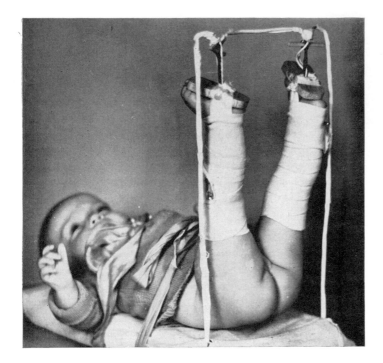

FIG. 178. Bryant traction may be mounted on a board. A foam rubber pad and a restraint about the torso are added. Rubber bands suspend the feet. The child is easily cared for and can be transported.

FIG. 179. N. S., female, age 5. Ischemic necrosis is a catastrophic complication of Bryant's traction. Double overhead traction for a fractured *right* femur brought on an acute ischemia in the *left* calf as is frequently the case. With pain, pallor, and paralysis of the toes, bandages must be loosened at once and traction removed if necessary. With appropriate cast and brace treatment, the deformity of the left foot disappeared and function returned almost to normal. The end result is not always so fortunate.

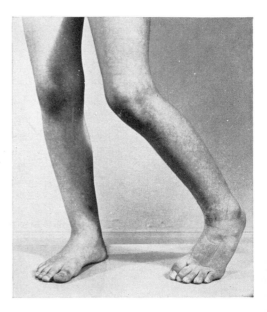

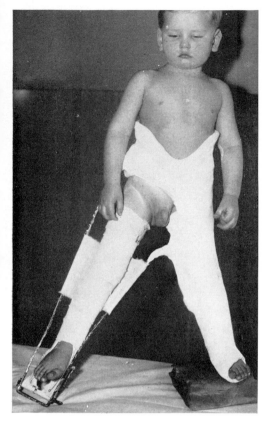

FIG. 180. Traction in abduction with well leg countertraction by means of a Hoke cast is ideal for the transportation of children with fractures of the femur who are too old to be suspended on a board. Constant traction is maintained by the ratchet at the end of the bars. Sometimes the affected leg is partially included in plaster. Traction eliminates pain and prevents angulation of the fragments. This device may be used for trochanteric fractures. [Reproduced with permission of Southern Medical Journal (87).]

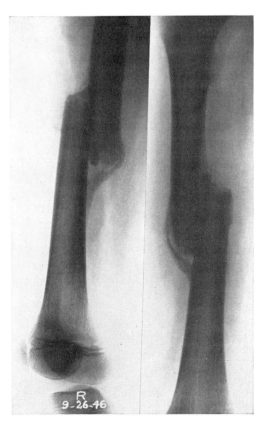

FIG. 181. R. L., male, age 8, 9/26/46. Roentgenogram five weeks after a fracture of the right femur. Alignment is perfect but overriding is excessive.

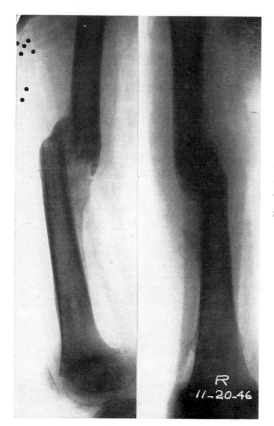

FIG. 182. R. L. The union shown in Figure 181 was easily broken up under anesthesia. With skeletal traction, the overriding was reduced to 1 cm. Thirteen weeks after the fracture, union was again solid.

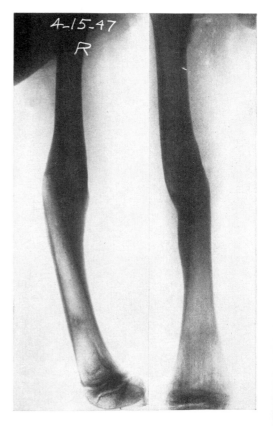

FIG. 183. R. L., 4/15/47, six months after the fracture. The position and the length were satisfactory then but there had been a tremendous stimulation to longitudinal growth. Two years later the right femur was 6 mm. too long and the right tibia was 7 mm. too long. In a case of this type, overriding of 2 cm. should have been permitted to remain. With stapling of the right femur, the inequality was corrected.

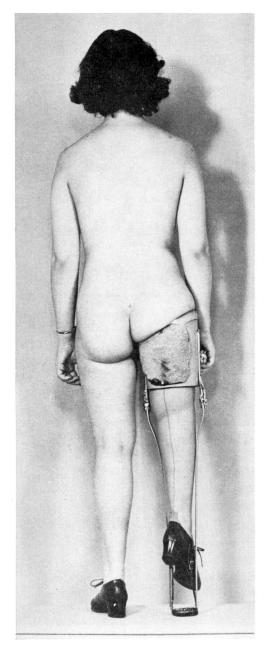

FIG. 184. V. S., female, age 21. The end result of a closed fracture of the middle of the right femur treated by open reduction and plating at the age of six. The resulting nonunion was unsuccessfully treated by four bone grafts. The roentgenographic appearance is shown in Figure 185. [Reproduced with permission of the Southern Medical Journal (87).]

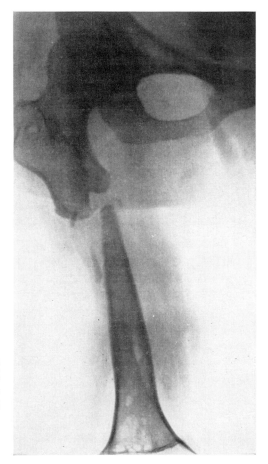

FIG. 185. V. S. The catastrophic end result of an unnecessary open reduction and plating. The girl would have been better with an amputation. [Reproduced with permission of the Southern Medical Journal (87).]

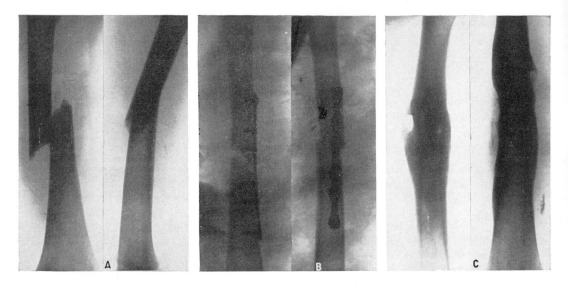

FIG. 186. R. M., male, age 8. A. 7/21/29. Closed fracture of the left femur would have given a perfect end result if allowed to remain in this position. B. 7/29/29. End to end apposition was the goal of the surgeon who performed an open operation and applied a Lane plate. The plate and screws were removed ten weeks later and in another month a sequestrectomy was performed because of infection. C. 6/22/31. Saucerization was necessary two years after the fracture. Five years after the fracture the quadriceps mechanism was lengthened. There was permanent disability. [Reproduced with permission of the Southern Medical Journal (87).]

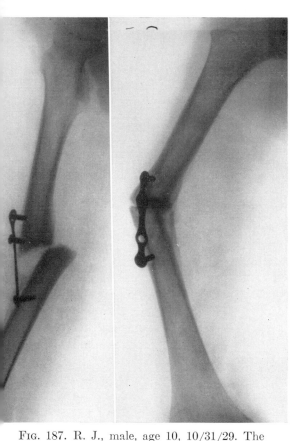

FIG. 187. R. J., male, age 10, 10/31/29. The right femur was fractured five months before this roentgenogram. After two weeks of traction perfect end to end apposition was not obtained. An open reduction and a very poor plating job were done. The surgeon's judgment was apparently on a par with his technical ability. In a cast, union occurred. Refracture on removal of the cast. The hardware was removed and a second cast applied. There was a refracture one year after removing it. Two years later there was a third refracture necessitating a cast for four months. The patient wore a brace for three years until the femur was solid enough to permit unsupported weight bearing. The left femur was small, atrophic and 4 mm. short. The scar of two operations was adherent to bone. Years of needless invalidism were caused by an unnecessary operation.

FIG. 188. L. P., female, age 11, 10/22/47. The left femur of this eleven year old girl was broken two years previously. The unnecessary insertion of the queer hardware was followed by angular deformity, overgrowth, coxa vara, and a draining sinus. On admission the left femur was 5 mm. short. After removal of the hardware, subsidence of the infection, and completion of a subtrochanteric osteotomy to correct the coxa vara, the left femur was 15 mm. too long. Further temporary acceleration of growth was expected. Staples were inserted in the distal end of the left femur and left in situ until the legs were of equal length. Following removal of the staples, continued growth proceeded symmetrically.

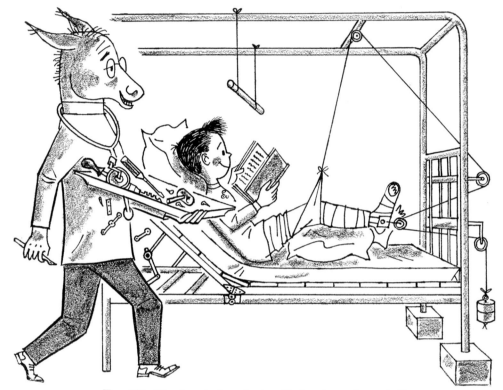

Fig. 189. The boy is fine, doctor. No hardware is needed!

Injuries at the Proximal End of the Femur

A thrust in the long axis of the thigh particularly with the femur in a distorted position will occasionally produce a fracture of the neck of the femur, or a traumatic epiphyseal separation (Figs. 190–193). The record should show clearly the differentiation from a pathologic epiphyseal displacement (adolescent coxa vara) which is discussed later. True fractures at the proximal end of the femur are so rare that no one has a great experience with them. They are usually indifferently treated with bad results (Figs. 194 to 197). The published reports (88, 89, 90, 91) show that the great hazard is avascular necrosis with resultant deformity and disability during adult life. Some men have obtained good results with closed reduction and a cast. This treatment is more likely to succeed in epiphyseal fractures (Fig. 191) than in those through the middle of the neck. If necessary, for accurate reduction and efficient immobilization, prompt internal fixation is justified in this difficult fracture. The usual Smith-Petersen nail is too large for use in the neck of a femur of a young child. One-eighth inch (3 mm.) adjustable nails are entirely satisfactory. Injury of the epiphyseal plate is unlikely from transfixion with two or three such pins, and longitudinal growth should continue. Premature closure is assured, however, and the case should be followed until growth is complete.

Slipped femoral epiphysis (adolescent coxa vara) is a disorder of both sexes, much more common in the male. It usually appears at puberty, but may occur as early as ten. Most of the patients are of the flabby fat type with retarded sexual development and obvious glandular dysfunction. An occasional one is a lean, physically active, sexually precocious adolescent. The early symptoms of pain in the knee or hip, and limp may exist for many months before the disability is sufficient to bring the patient to the doctor. Then, too often, the examination is limited to the knee because the pain is referred there. It is imperative that physicians who treat fractures in children and adolescents become familiar with the symptoms, findings, and treatment of this entity.

The patient walks with a limp on the affected side with the foot externally rotated, the hip adducted. He has a positive Trendelenburg sign on this side. Physical examination at this time shows restriction of all motions of the affected hip, but particularly of abduction and rotation inward. If posterior slipping has progressed to a considerable degree, extension may be abnormally increased, while flexion is limited.

The roentgenogram in the anteroposterior projection will frequently show widening of the transluscent zone of the epiphyseal plate due to displacement of the caput, but more often this zone is obscured by superimposition. Slipping of the epiphysis is usually, but not always, associated

with some coxa vara (Fig. 198). The lateral view of the neck in the Lauenstein position (Fig. 201) is usually more revealing than the anteroposterior
view (Fig. 199), particularly in the early case (Fig. 202). The diagnosis
should be made when the symptoms first appear.

The *treatment* is conservative and/or operative. Conservative management includes preliminary bed rest with traction in the longitudinal axis
of the limb as well as in internal rotation in combination with medical
management of the hypoglandularism, if present. In the case without
complete separation of the caput, muscle spasm will disappear rapidly and
a considerable degree of actual correction of the deformity may be obtained. The hip must be protected for a prolonged period. If the caput has
been suddenly completely separated, reduction is easily accomplished by
the same method of traction. In either case, the hip is vulnerable until the
epiphysis has fused. Aggravation of pre-existing symptoms or an acute
separation may occur when activity is resumed. For this reason, one is
justified in the primary operative treatment of a slipped femoral epiphysis
if an experienced orthopaedic surgeon and a first class operating theater
are available. The operative indications change with (1) the chronicity of
the disease (duration and amount of slipping), and (2) the recentness of
the complete separation, when it occurs. The following table gives these
indications in outline form.

Conservative treatment (92) is used temporarily in adolescent coxa
vara (slipped femoral epiphysis), or because operative treatment is not
available.

Operative treatment of various stages of the disease

I. Incomplete separation of caput and metaphysis.

    A. Minimal slip of caput on metaphysis (less than 1 cm.) (93)
        (1) Unfused epiphyseal plate—fixation with nails.
        (2) Fused epiphyseal plate—no treatment necessary.
    B. Moderate slip of caput on metaphysis (about 1 cm.)
        (1) Unfused epiphyseal plate—fixation with nails and simultaneous oste-
            otomy (4, 74) (Fig. 202).
        (2) Fused epiphyseal plate—subtrochanteric osteotomy without nailing.
    C. Extreme slip of caput posterior on metaphysis (over 1 cm.)
        (1) Unfused—open operation with separation at epiphyseal plate, re-
            duction, and nailing; or wedge osteotomy of the neck, reduction, and
            nailing.
        (2) Fused.
            (a) Good motion—wedge osteotomy of the neck, reduction, and
                nailing.
            (b) Only 30° total range of hip motion. Unilateral—with pain on
                motion— arthrodesis. Bilateral—arthroplasty, displacement oste-

otomy, prosthesis or other palliative operation on one or both hips selected according to age, sex, and occupation. In male, an arthrodesis on one side is often desirable.

II. With sudden complete separation of caput and metaphysis.
    A. Early in disease, minimal neck changes.
        (1) Fresh separation—closed reduction and nailing.
        (2) Four weeks old—wedge resection, open reduction and nailing.
    B. Late in the disease (deformity of the neck established)
        (1) Fresh separation—wedge resection of the neck, open reduction and nailing (Fig. 200).
        (2) Four weeks old—same treatment as B (1).
        (3) Ancient.
            (a) Good motion—same treatment as B (1).
            (b) Only 30° total range of hip motion. Unilateral—arthrodesis. Bilateral—arthroplasty, displacement osteotomy, or prosthesis, or other palliative operation on one or both hips. In a male, an arthrodesis on one side is often desirable.

In maintaining the position of the caput on the metaphysis of the femur, three ⅛″ (3 mm.) adjustable nails are usually preferable to a single trifin nail. The latter is designed to traverse the neck of an atrophic adult femur. Here it is an efficient unit. When two dense surfaces of bone are to be held from slipping it is less effective than three widely dispersed nails. It is particularly clumsy when there is considerable displacement. The slender nails may be crossed within the neck so that they obtain a good hold on the thicker portion of the caput. A single trifin nail must necessarily aim at the cephalad and anterior portion of the epiphysis, which is very thin with very little margin of safety. Often it must be driven through the posterior cortex of the neck in order to reach its goal. There is less trauma associated with drilling in three small caliber nails than with driving of a composite nail through the exceedingly hard metaphyseal zone. This means less likelihood of injury to the blood supply, and less danger of subsequent avascular necrosis.

Pinning alone is the method of choice even when the caput has slipped as much as 1 cm. When the deformity is sufficient to justify osteotomy in the stage of continued slipping, then pinning may be combined with subtrochanteric osteotomy to obtain more abduction, internal rotation, and flexion of the distal fragment (Fig. 202).

The moderate slips with fused epiphyseal plates which have become painfree with residual deformity are best corrected by a subtrochanteric osteotomy (4). Coxa vara may be fully corrected. The operation is contraindicated only when the posterior displacement of the head is exceedingly great. The operation is rarely followed by avascular necrosis and is much safer than a direct attack upon the neck of the femur. It often eliminates the limp and establishes a very satisfactory range of motion.

Wedge osteotomy of the neck of the femur at the metaphyseal zone with the base cephalad and anterior, is justified in the absence of complete separation, in the active stage and even after healing has begun, if the deformity is extreme. No other procedure is of value. The operation is a difficult one and must be performed with a minimum of trauma. It should not be attempted except under the direction of one who has performed the operation many times. While there is a definite risk of avascular necrosis of the femoral head, the incidence is even greater with cast fixation alone, or with attempted forced manipulation and cast fixation. The latter combination is rarely successful even temporarily, and almost invariably eventuates in a stiff hip.

With minimal trauma or none at all, the capital epiphysis may separate completely off the neck in either the early or late stage of the disease. If seen promptly in the early stage there is no doubt that gentle closed reduction followed by blind nailing gives an excellent result in most cases. If the separation occurs suddenly in a late stage of the disease with existing marked deformity of the neck and eburnation of the exposed portion of the metaphysis, then manipulative reduction replaces the capital epiphysis only in the position of deformity where it was before the final slip and not in its normal position. The manipulation has served only to endanger further the blood supply of the capital epiphysis. In such a case, primary wedge resection of the cephalad portion of the neck, gentle curettement of the epiphyseal surface of the head, and accurate replacement in the normal position, is the operation of choice. This is not as hazardous as a wedge osteotomy in the ancient case which has not completely separated. In such a case, all of the trauma of the osteotomy is transmitted to the head. When the head has already separated spontaneously, and an anvil retractor (94) is slipped under the neck, the osteotomy can be performed without any trauma being transmitted to the head. Once the neck is cut away, the head may be replaced, still without trauma, by inward rotation and abduction of the shaft. In the hands of an expert, this operation yields a high percentage of good results.

In the treatment of slipped femoral epiphysis, the high incidence of bilaterality (20 per cent to 40 per cent) must be recognized. In some clinics, the appearance of the disorder in one hip is considered an indication to nail both hips (95). A less radical approach is to examine both hips clinically and by roentgenograms at the time of the first visit. If the second hip is normal, the parents are warned that it may become similarly involved at any time. Very often the child is brought in within a year to have the second hip nailed. Prompt treatment is needed to prevent the complete slip which greatly complicates the problem. The parents must understand this fully.

Congenital coxa vara, sometimes wrongly designated *congenital fracture of the neck of the femur* is a developmental anomaly of one or both hips characterized by shortening, limited abduction, and a roentgenogram showing a varus position of the neck of the femur. In the infant or young child the middle portion of the neck may be entirely cartilaginous so that the appearance is suggestive of a fracture (Fig. 203). Bone grafting has been done to "secure union". It is superfluous. Subtrochanteric osteotomy with blade plate fixation in the young child (Fig. 204), leads to prompt ossification of the cartilage zone and correction of the limp. If the varus is extreme, it may be corrected in two or even three stages to avoid sacrificing length.

Traumatic dislocation of the hip is exceedingly rare in young children (Fig. 205). Reports in the literature are mostly of isolated cases (97, 98, 99). In adolescents, it is less likely to be complicated by a fracture of the acetabulum than in adults. The diagnosis of the posterior dislocation (70 per cent) can be made from the position of the extremity in internal rotation and flexion (Fig. 207), as contrasted to the shortening and external rotation of fracture of the neck of the femur (Fig. 208). A roentgenogram is necessary for the record.

Reduction of the posterior dislocation is accomplished under general anesthesia with the least trauma by flexing the thigh to a right angle and lifting the flexed knee toward the ceiling, in adduction. The thigh is abducted and extended only after the femoral head slips into place. The same maneuver will convert an anterior dislocation to a posterior one and then reduce it. The historic violent reduction methods by apparatus or levering against the "Y" ligament were developed in the absence of anesthesia. They are exceedingly traumatic. Open reduction is unnecessary unless treatment has been delayed for two weeks. After two or three months an angulation osteotomy (4) will give a better ultimate result than an open reduction followed by fibrous ankylosis. Arthrodesis in good position is an acceptable outcome in the male, but is not better than the osteotomy if the length of the legs is equalized.

Avascular necrosis is a less common sequel than in adults but when it occurs the end result is even more devastating. For this reason a dislocated hip should be protected from full weight bearing for three months. If there is no evidence of avascular necrosis by that time, it is unlikely, but delayed osteochondral changes much like those of coxa plana do occur (100).

Trochanteric fractures are also prone to develop avascular necrosis of the caput. A hip spica with wide abduction for eight weeks will usually immobilize the fragments adequately. The *subcervical fracture* is one that is likely to heal in the varus position, and it should be operated upon in most cases (Fig. 195). A child size blade plate is used to restore and maintain the normal angle.

It is true that angular deformities below the lesser trochanter straighten out with growth, but when trochanteric and subtrochanteric fractures heal with a coxa vara deformity (Figs. 209, 210), the loss of the neck angle is permanent in spite of molding, as discussed in Chapter I (Fig. 211).

The short proximal fragment of a subtrochanteric fracture is pulled into flexion by the psoas (Fig. 212) while the hip extensors act more strongly on the distal fragment. The temptation to do an open reduction in a child should be resisted. In young children and sometimes in older ones, accurate reduction may be obtained by acutely flexing both hips with overhead traction. If Russell traction is used in an older child, an additional sling may be placed under the knee of the affected side to produce more acute angulation at the hip and knee (Fig. 214). When the distal fragment has been brought in line with the flexed proximal fragment, the position can be maintained by continued traction. Bayonet apposition is permissible and even desirable in the displaced fracture. Slight angulation is acceptable in a young child (Fig. 213). One must be careful to avoid excessive angulation with the apex laterally which produces permanent coxa vara (Fig. 210).

In a *high fracture of the shaft*, the short proximal fragment may be abducted from loss of adductor pull. The alignment is corrected by increasing the traction on the affected extremity in the abducted position. In the low fracture of the upper third, as in one of the middle third, an adducted proximal fragment is aligned by lessening the pull on the affected leg and adding more traction to the opposite leg so as to abduct the pelvis to the side of the fracture (Fig. 172). The need for close supervision of traction cannot be overemphasized. Failures are due to the way the method is applied rather than to any fault with the method itself. Van Eden (101) observed that the traction treatment of fractures of the femur in children was better in small hospitals where the attending surgeon personally supervised the entire treatment than in the large hospitals where treatment was left to the house officers. This should not be true if the residents are trained in the principles of fracture management.

Avulsion fracture of the greater trochanter may occur as an isolated injury or may be associated with dislocation of the hip (Fig. 215). The simple avulsion heals promptly with the leg immobilized in abduction. *Avulsion of the lesser trochanter* is the result of muscular violence. It heals with displacement but little or no disability.

Fractures of the Distal End of the Femur

Forced hyperextension of the knee may produce an epiphyseal separation of the distal end of the femur (Fig. 216) with gross displacement; the wagon wheel injury of the horse and buggy days. If the injury is seen promptly, accurate closed reduction usually offers no problem under general anesthesia. Once the fracture is reduced there is no tendency to displacement (102). A long cast with the knee in slight flexion will immobilize the fracture until union is solid in three to four weeks.

If reduction is delayed, it may be very difficult. Occasionally this fracture becomes a surgical emergency because the metaphyseal fragment protrudes against the popliteal vessels (103). If there is circulatory embarrassment and the fracture cannot be easily reduced by closed methods, prompt open operation is indicated (104). Legs have been lost through delay.

An epiphyseal separation should be accurately reduced in most cases, but with moderate displacement and good alignment it will heal without loss of function. In a child under ten, angulation of 10° to 20° with the apex posterior will cause no significant back knee and only temporary loss of flexion. Angulation with the apex anterior will cause prolonged flexion. Knock knee and bow leg deformities diminish only slightly with growth.

Supracondylar fractures of the femur just above the epiphyseal plate are rare. They may be treated in traction with the knee and hip flexed at right angles (Fig. 214). In young children when there is difficulty holding the fragment it is occasionally expedient to immobilize the knee in acute flexion. The fracture is analogous to the supracondylar fracture of the elbow and may be similarly treated. The same care must be taken to watch the circulation.

The *"T" fractures of the femoral condyles* so frequently encountered in adults are exceedingly rare in children. They may be treated with traction below the knee. A Kirschner wire through the tibial crest may be used if necessary. The soft parts serve to hold the fragments in fair apposition. Considerable displacement of a supracondylar fracture is permissible. Bayonet apposition is acceptable in a young child, but alignment should be reasonably good.

Oblique fractures through the distal femoral epiphysis are usually the result of direct violence. Anatomic reduction is not necessary. The management may be difficult enough to justify a Kirschner wire through the crest of the tibia. A long leg cast with the knee flexed should stabilize the wire. Open operation will increase the likelihood of epiphyseal damage.

The prognosis is good in most distal femoral *epiphyseal displacements* of adolescents. Premature closure of the epiphyseal plate usually occurs, but there is rarely more than a few millimeters difference in leg length. Fractures produced by great violence with injury of the growing cells of the epiphyseal plate, whether they are incomplete, transverse, or oblique, are likely to be complicated by retarded growth with both linear and angular deformity (Figs. 217, 218). Prompt recognition of the epiphyseal damage and appropriate treatment are imperative if permanent disability is to be avoided. Repeated osteotomies are necessary in a young child to correct the angulation and at the same time accelerate growth of the damaged bone. Sometimes a wedge or "napkin-ring" of bone from the bank may be inserted, but one must be careful not to extend the host bone too much. Skin sloughs, and more serious complications have occurred. Internal fixation is desirable in the older child. Growth of the opposite femur should be retarded promptly by stapling, but not before eight years (Fig. 219). An angular deformity in a short bone should not be corrected by stapling. In the treatment of deformities from epiphyseal injury, it is imperative that one understand the rates of growth (Fig. 147, p. 106) of the various epiphyses which have been computed from actuarial studies (105). It is also necessary to know the time of closure of the epiphyses (Figs. 1 and 2, pp. 4, 5). Variations may be anticipated by obtaining an accurate growth history of the progenitors.

Treatment of fractures of the femur in children in the past has been lacking in appreciation of the late sequelae. Each patient must be followed until one can be sure that there will be no inequality of leg length. The surgeon who treats such deformities must keep as his goal, the ideal appearance and function of the extremities when the children are through growing.

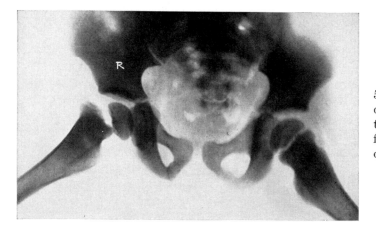

FIG. 190. I. K., male, age 4, 5/21/29. A fall from a fire escape caused this traumatic separation of the proximal epiphysis of the right femur. [Reproduced with permission of Southern Medical Journal (87).

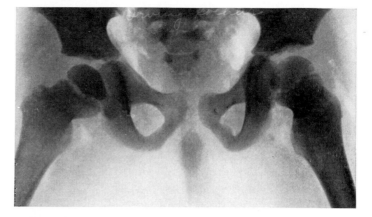

FIG. 191. I. K., 8/1/29. The fracture was reduced under anesthesia and immobilized in plaster for eight weeks. Note the relative increased density of the right capital epiphysis at ten weeks. Unfortunately the boy was not prevented from weight bearing. [Reproduced with permission of the Southern Medical Journal (87).]

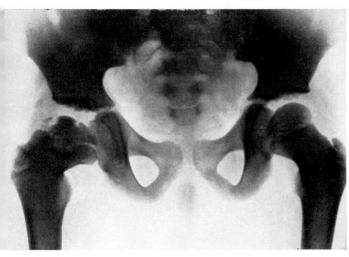

FIG. 192. I. K., 12/11/30, seven months after the fracture. Avascular necrosis of the capital epiphysis had already appeared. Weight bearing was continued. [Reproduced with permission of the Southern Medical Journal (87).]

FIG. 193. I. K., 5/4/35, six years after the fracture. Revascularization had occurred but with deformity which would have been prevented had weight bearing been eliminated. In the next seven years the varus deformity of the right hip increased. [Reproduced with permission of the Southern Medical Journal (87).]

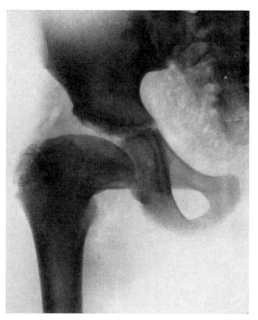

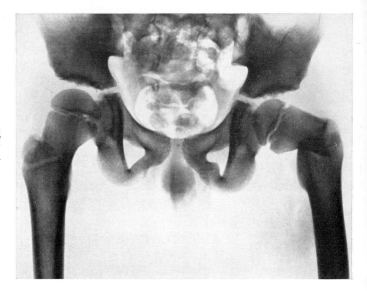

FIG. 194. R. S. P., male, age 5, 1/7/51. A subcervical fracture of the left femur caused by a toboggan accident.

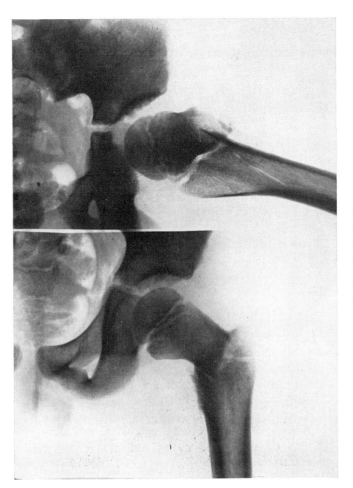

FIG. 195. R. S. P., 1/30/51. After traction in bed for two weeks the antero-posterior roentgenogram did not look too bad but the lateral view showed gross displacement. Further reduction was not attempted. The boy was allowed to walk with crutches.

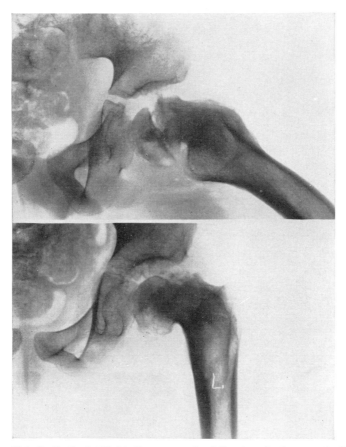

FIG. 196. R. S. P., 8/15/51. Seven months following the fracture in Figure 194, there were coxa vara, epiphysiolysis, and avascular necrosis of the capital epiphysis. Adduction, flexion, external rotation deformity were extreme and the limp was grotesque.

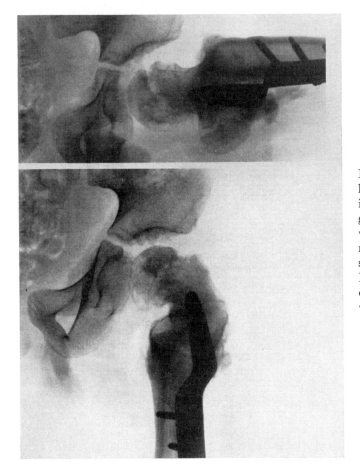

FIG. 197. R. S. P., 10/24/52. Fourteen months following an angulation, rotation osteotomy with internal fixation. Function was greatly improved. The hardware was removed at this time. The right distal femoral epiphysis was stapled to equalize leg length. Motion of the left hip remained considerably restricted but the boy walked with scarcely a limp.

FIG. 198. R. H., male, age 14, 1/28/42. Sudden separation of the right capital epiphysis after six months of limping. Note the chronic changes in the metaphysis. This was a pathologic, not an acute traumatic fracture.

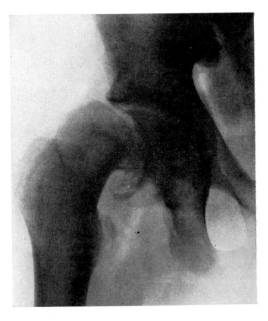

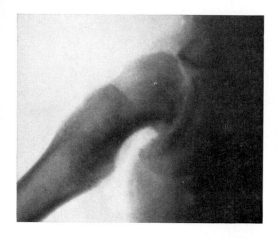

Fig. 199. R. H., 1/28/42. A lateral view of the hip shown in Figure 198. The deposition of bone on the posterior margin of the metaphysis was clearly shown. There was an acute complete separation of a femoral epiphysis engrafted on a chronic slipping.

Fig. 200. R. H., 1/12/42. Antero posterior and lateral views of the same hip shown in Figure 199 following wedge resection of the metaphysis, open reduction, and nailing of the capital epiphysis in normal position. An excellent result was obtained. The nails were later removed.

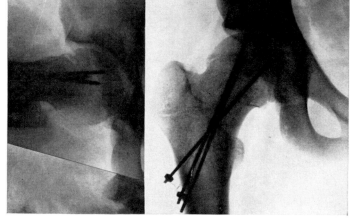

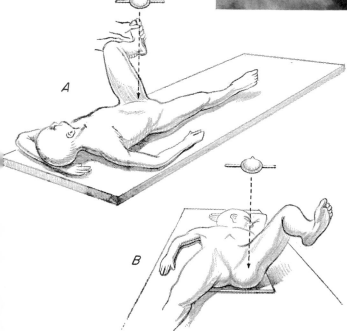

Fig. 201. A lateral view of the proximal end of the femur is best obtained by the Lauenstein position with 45° flexion and 45° abduction as shown. The tube is centered directly over the capital epiphysis. The femoral head and neck are shown in profile. See Figure 202.

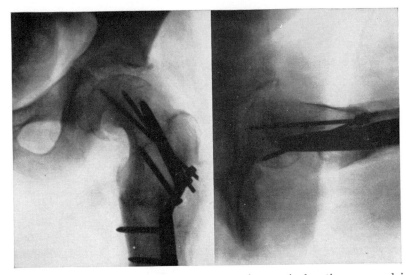

FIG. 202. A. S., male, age 13, 12/12/42. Limp of a year's duration was explained by moderate slipping of the capital epiphysis without acute separation. There was coxa vara in the anteroposterior view and posterior displacement of the capital epiphysis in the lateral view. Internal rotation and abduction were limited. The roentgenogram was taken eight weeks following a subtrochanteric osteotomy with internal fixation. The coxa vara was corrected by angulation, apex medially and the rotation, by inward torsion of the distal fragment. Further slipping was prevented by the simultaneous insertion of two adjustable nails. [Reproduced with permission of the Journal of Bone and Joint Surgery (74).]

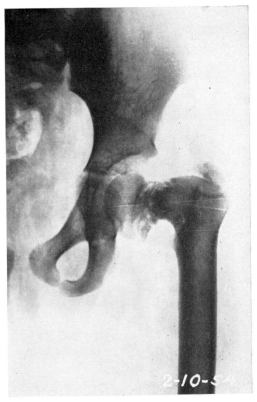

FIG. 203. R. K., female, age 5. Congenital coxa vara of the left hip, sometimes improperly called "congenital fracture of the neck of the femur". The abnormality was associated with limp. Abduction limited 40°, internal rotation limited 25°; external rotation 50° in excess of normal. Early correction of this deformity was desirable.

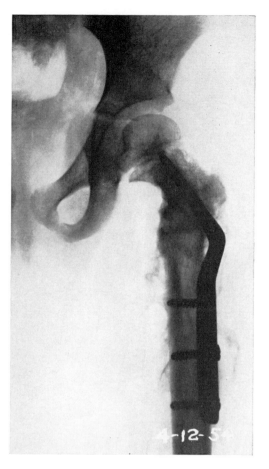

FIG. 204. R. K., the same case as Figure 203, seven weeks after an osteotomy to correct the angulation and rotation. Internal fixation was secure and a cast unnecessary. A bone graft would have been superfluous. The cartilage islands which gave the appearance of a fracture readily disappeared when the weight bearing thrust was corrected. The blade plate and screws were removed in six months.

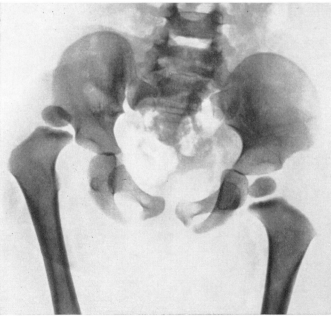

FIG. 205. E. W., female, age 21 months, 3/1/52. Roentgenogram immediately after an automobile backed over her. No injury other than superficial abrasions and posterior dislocation of the left hip. Closed reduction under general anesthesia. Plaster immobilization for five weeks. She started weight bearing fourteen weeks after the injury. The child limped occasionally during the first year, but recovered completely. (Courtesy of Dr. F. H. Foreman.)

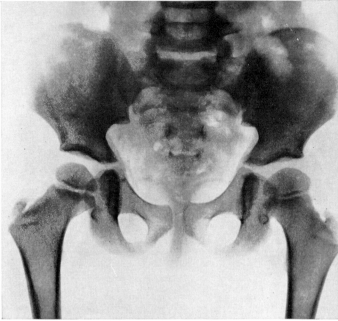

FIG. 206. E. W., 4/19/54, roentgenogram following figure 205, two
years after the closed reduction.
The child was clinically well and
had a bilaterally negative Trendelenburg sign. (Courtesy of Dr. F. H.
Foreman.)

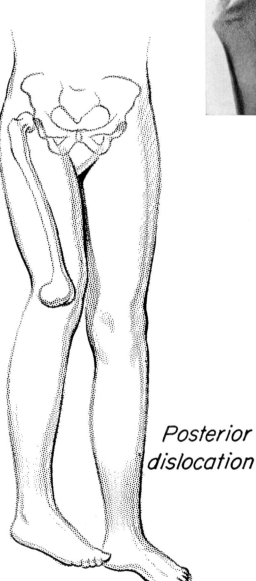

*Posterior
dislocation*

FIG. 207. The right leg is in the characteristic
position assumed with a posterior dislocation of the
hip; shortening with internal rotation and flexion
Compare with Figure 208.

Fracture of femur

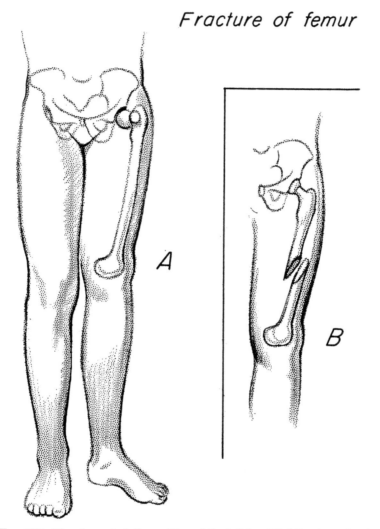

FIG. 208. The characteristic position of the left leg (A) following a fracture of the neck of the femur with shortening, external rotation and with the trochanter riding high, (B) with fracture of the shaft of the femur. the leg externally rotated but the relations of the hip remain normal.

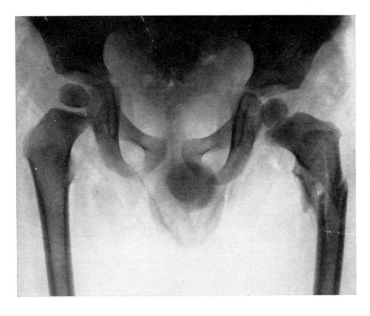

Fig. 209. J. H., male, age 26 months, 2/7/53. Comminuted trochanteric and subtrochanteric fractures of the left femur in an automobile collision. Treatment with Bryant's traction. (Courtesy of Dr. R. S. Rilling.)

Fig. 210. J. H., 5/15/54. Healing of the preceding fracture in coxa vara with 15 mm. shortening. This is a disabling deformity that will require correction by osteotomy. Such a fracture is best treated by wide abduction. This may be obtained by a cast or traction or both (Fig. 180). Courtesy of Dr. R. S. Rilling.)

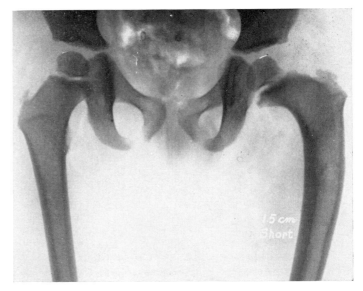

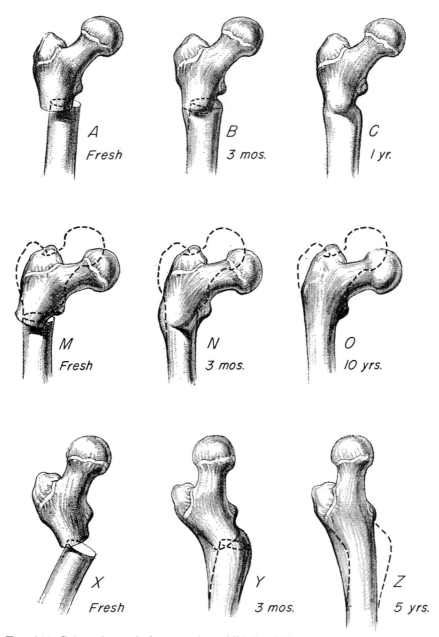

FIG. 211. Subtrochanteric fractures in a child should be normally aligned. A. bayonet apposition is satisfactory. B. Molding takes care of the local deformity. Slight flexion of the proximal fragment is permissible. Moderate overriding is equalized by accelerated growth. In one year, function should be normal. M. Angulation into coxa vara is not permissible. N. Coxa vara remains as a permanent deformity. There is no change in the neck angle as a result of growth. O. The local irregularity disappears but the coxa vara remains. X. Conversely, a subtrochanteric osteotomy to correct coxa vara is permanently effective. Y. The angle between the neck and the long axis remains constant. Z. The subtrochanteric angular protrusion gradually disappears. If the operation was performed to stabilize a dislocated hip, then its effectiveness gradually diminishes and the angulation osteotomy must be repeated.

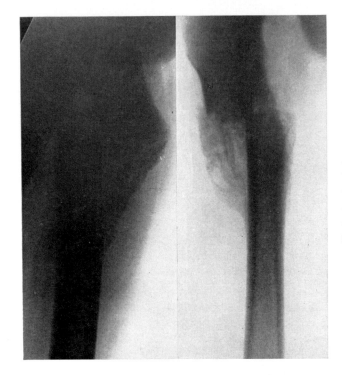

FIG 212. H. T., male, age 7, 1/26/34. With traction this subtrochanteric fracture healed with bayonet apposition. In the lateral view (on the left) there was flexion of the proximal fragment. This could have been eliminated by flexing the hip.

FIG. 213. H. T. Six years after the preceding figure the local deformity had been obliterated by molding. Alignment was now normal. Leg length was the same and motions of the hip were normal.

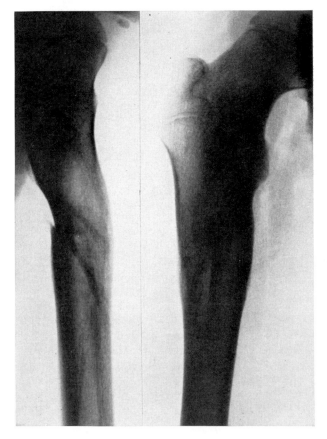

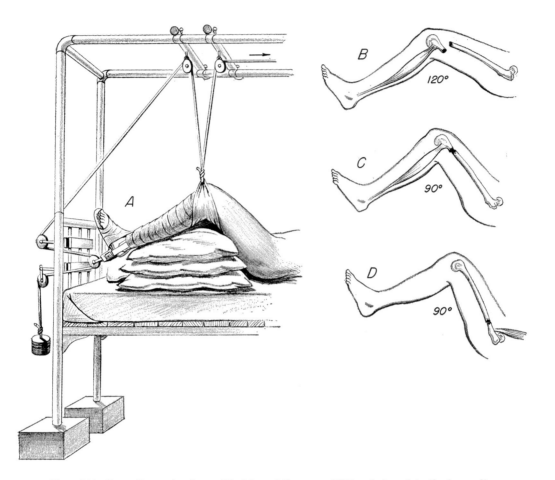

FIG. 214. Russell traction is modified by adding an additional strand to the knee sling and pulling upward. A. Care must be taken to avoid compressing the peroneal nerve. The sling must be soft without being too yielding. Felt in stockinet is a good combination. B. For supracondylar fractures of the femur, the additional flexion (C) will align the distal fragment with the proximal. D. In subtrochanteric fractures of the femur it is important to flex the hip by the same means. Here the lower leg is more nearly horizontal. The pulleys at the foot are raised, and more pillows placed under the leg.

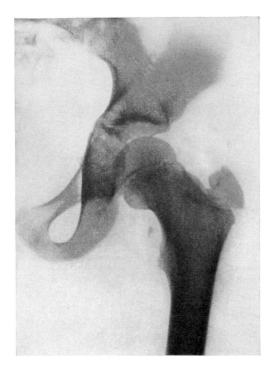

Fig. 215. D. H., male, age 8. In an automobile accident the left hip was dislocated and the greater and lesser trochanters avulsed. Reduction of the dislocation restored the trochanters to a reasonably good position. They united without deformity but the capital epiphysis went on to avascular necrosis. Contrast with Figures 205 and 206.

Fig. 216. J. S., male, age 15 Complete separation of the distal femoral epiphysis was reduced promptly under general anesthesia without difficulty. There were no complications. The distal femoral epiphysis on the right side closed a few months before the one on the left. There was 3 mm. of shortening. The length of the bones before the accident is not known. (Courtesy of Dr. Bruce Brewer.)

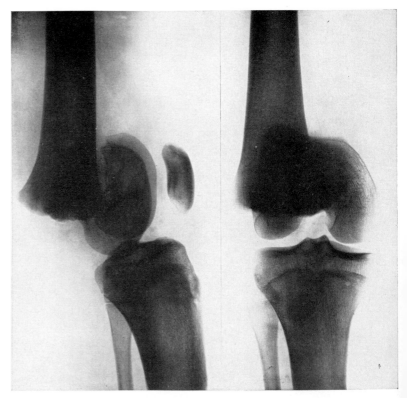

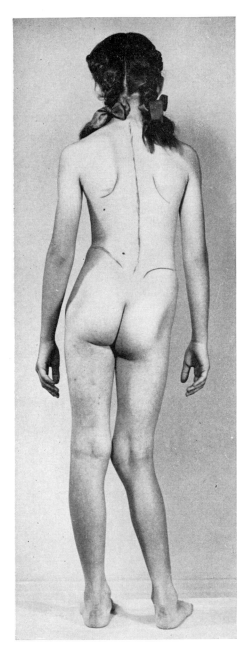

FIG. 217. F. K., female, age 9, 9/17/47. Seven years after a horse kicked her right knee injuring the distal femoral epiphysis, shortening and angular deformity were disabling as well as unsightly.

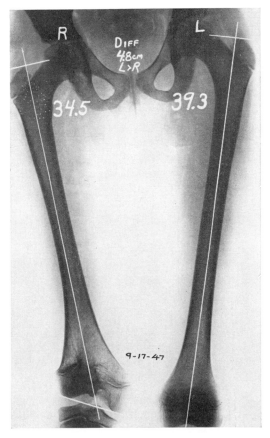

FIG. 218. F. K., the case shown in Figure 217. The central portion of the right distal femoral epiphyseal plate had been destroyed. Growth had been more retarded laterally than medially.

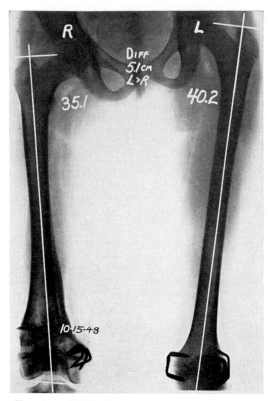

FIG. 219. F. K. Supracondylar osteotomy on the
right with insertion of a large block of bone from
the bank corrected the angulation. With this was
combined stapling of the medial side of the distal
femoral epiphysis. Usually multiple osteotomies are
preferable, but the parents were relatively tall.
The left distal femoral epiphysis was stapled to
retard growth of that bone.

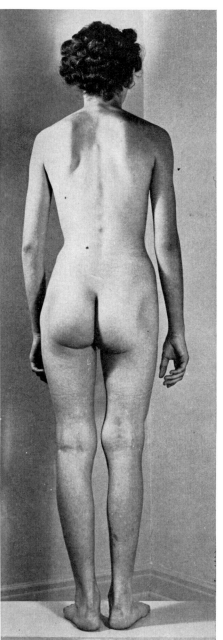

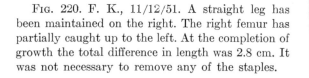

FIG. 220. F. K., 11/12/51. A straight leg has
been maintained on the right. The right femur has
partially caught up to the left. At the completion of
growth the total difference in length was 2.8 cm. It
was not necessary to remove any of the staples.

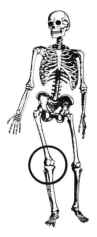

CHAPTER VIII

Fractures About the Knee

FRACTURES OF THE PATELLA

Transverse fractures of the patella are caused by a direct blow, by the indirect force of sudden violent flexion of the knee, or by a combination of the two. They occur much less frequently than in adults, because all of the tissues are more resilient. Following a previous injury, stiffness about the knee may predispose to such a fracture with a long tear of the extensor mechanism on either side (Fig. 221). As in the adult, an open reduction is necessary to repair the extensor mechanism. The bone fragments may be held in the normal position by a circular turn of wire about the patella (Fig. 222). The capsule is repaired with mattress sutures which are placed before the reduction and tied afterward. If secure fixation is not obtained, the patellar fragments will separate and form an elongated patella. Remember when interpreting roentgenograms that the peripheral portion of the patella is still cartilaginous.

Partite patellae may be confused with fractures of this bone in adolescents. The abnormality is usually present bilaterally. Comminuted fractures are rare and excision of the patella is unnecessary.

In a child the intact patella may be avulsed from the distal half of its normal fibrous covering in connection with a transverse rupture of the quadriceps mechanism. In such a case, the roentgenogram shows an upward riding patella and only a few flakes of bone adherent to the patellar ligament (Fig. 223). Replacement of the patella into its former location is accomplished like placing an egg in an egg cup (Fig. 224). Suture of the soft parts is sufficient. Plaster immobilization in extension for four weeks is desirable. Postoperative extension contractures do not occur in children, even if the immobilization is twice as long.

Avulsion of the anterior portion of the proximal tibial epiphysis is a rare injury of adolescence (106). Before the epiphysis has united at age seven-

171

teen to nineteen, the tonguelike anterior projection, or a larger portion may be torn loose and displaced upward by a violent extension of the knee. If the displacement is more than 1 or 2 mm., open reduction and suture or fixation with pins will be required to maintain the position of the loose fragment that has been carried upward by the patellar ligament. Following this injury in growing children, the prognosis should be guarded. Back knee due to premature closure of the anterior portion of the epiphysis is likely. Fortunately this injury occurs in older boys and the chance of gross deformity is slight.

Osgood-Schlatter's osteochondrosis of the tibial tuberosity (96) must be distinguished from a fracture. It occurs characteristically in boys thirteen or fourteen years old who have become active in violent sports. A tender bump appears just below the patellar ligament. The symptoms are usually unilateral although symmetrical lateral roentgenograms of the knees frequently show a bilateral irregularity of ossification of the tonguelike portion of the epiphysis. The diagnosis is made on the clinical findings. The roentgenogram is important in establishing the prognosis and planning treatment.

When the symptoms are of only a few month's duration and the roentgenogram is indicative of a simple inflammatory reaction of the epiphysis, the prognosis is good with plaster immobilization for six to eight weeks. The tenderness and bump will both disappear permanently. Drilling is superfluous and likely to lead to immediate epiphyseal closure, which is not desirable.

The case of long duration is likely to be confused with a fracture. A separate osseous center forms anteriorly. If treatment is delayed too long the separation becomes permanent and the bony enlargement is perpetuated by an ossicle which lies in a nest of granulation and/or fibrous tissue. The bump and the tender "nonunion" make kneeling painful or impossible (Fig. 225). When the symptoms of Osgood-Schlatter's disease are associated with the formation of this definite ossicle, much time will be saved by excising not only the ossicle but the bed.

The patellar ligament is split longitudinally and the two halves elevated to either side by sharp dissection without disturbing the peripheral attachment of the ligament. The entire prominence is removed with a large gouge. The cut does not go deep enough to endanger the epiphyseal plate. The halves of the patellar ligament are sutured together and the knee immobilized in plaster for three weeks. Prompt and permanent relief of the symptoms is afforded.

Avulsion of the Tibial Spine

Torsion strain combined with hyperextension of the knee of a child will avulse the attachment of the anterior cruciate ligament more frequently than in an adult. There is hemarthrosis and if the bone fragment is displaced, the knee cannot be fully extended. The symptoms are similar to those of a locked semilunar cartilage. The true nature of the injury should be suspected, because semilunar cartilage tears are exceedingly rare in children. A roentgenogram will show a thin flake of bone raised from the tibial plateau (Fig. 226). The differential diagnosis between this condition and osteochondrosis dissecans or chip fracture of the articular surface should not be difficult. Avulsion of the anterior cruciate usually occurs in children between six and twelve years, while the other two occur after that age.

If the injury is recognized promptly, arthrotomy through an anterior incision will permit accurate replacement of the fragment. It is held in position by a loop of wire through the anterior cruciate ligament at its attachment, over the fragment, and down through drill holes in the front of the proximal tibial epiphysis. The trick is to drill two holes that converge slightly to the medial and lateral margins of the defect. A separate loop of wire is passed upward through each drill hole. An end of the first wire is caught with each loop and pulled down through the corresponding hole. The ends of the wire are twisted together or tied just distal to the tibial tuberosity (Fig. 227). Great care must be taken not to damage the epiphyseal cartilage which should lie entirely distal and posterior to the holes. After six or eight weeks, the wire is easily removed. The end result should be perfect. If the epiphyseal cartilage is damaged, a back knee will result.

If the fracture has been neglected for two or three weeks and/or the fragment is not grossly displaced (Fig. 228), a better result will be obtained with conservative treatment. A cast should be applied with the knee in 10° less than complete extension for three or four weeks. Roentgenograms will show a bump on the tibial plateau, but function is surprisingly good immediately and eventually it will be entirely normal (Fig. 229).

Chip Fractures of the Femoral Condyle

Athletic injuries of adolescents, particularly from football and basketball occasionally combine flexion of the knee with a direct blow so as to chip off a piece of bone and cartilage from the femoral condyle, rarely the patella. Symptoms of internal derangement of the knee appear immediately. There is hemarthrosis and great disability. Usually the knee cannot be fully extended; occasionally it cannot be flexed. Intermittent locking may develop. Carefully positioned roentgenograms will disclose a paperthin flake of bone (Fig. 230).

The diagnosis is sometimes difficult. The exact origin of the bone is rarely seen on a roentgenogram (Fig. 231), and sometimes the defect cannot be seen at operation without a large exploratory incision, which is not justified.

Prompt arthrotomy should be performed for removal of the loose piece. The roentgenographic shadow is no indication of its size. A thin layer of osseous granules is attached to a full thickness piece of articular cartilage. Spontaneous repair of the defect is usually complete. Unless removal of the free body has been delayed (Fig. 231), the prognosis is good for normal function even if the injury borders on a weight bearing surface.

A differential diagnosis between this chip fracture and a true osteochondrosis dissecans is necessary for insurance or medicolegal reasons. The fracture comes on without prodromes and is the result of a sudden violent injury. Disability is immediate and complete. Osteochondrosis dissecans will usually grumble for several weeks. In this early stage, roentgenograms will disclose the piece of bone and cartilage still in situ (Fig. 232), surrounded by a zone of rarefaction on the lateral aspect of the medial condyle of the femur. Only if the loose fragment has become displaced as a free body, is operation indicated. In the early stages, the sequestrated body will revascularize if not molested. A plaster cast for six to eight weeks has permitted complete healing in most cases. Conservative treatment should not be abandoned unless the fragment is actually displaced. All too frequently an operation has been performed only to find the cartilage surface intact. Do not remove the roentgenologically demarcated body in a child unless there is a break in the cartilage. Drilling is superfluous in view of the excellent results that are obtained with simple conservative measures. It is unwise in the late case when partial separation has already occurred. Operation should then include removal of the dead piece of bone and cartilage and smoothing of the edges of the crater. Healing of the defect with a fibro-cartilaginous scar gives a satisfactory end result, but not as perfect as the one obtained by conservative measures when the case is seen earlier.

Tears of the semilunar cartilages are rare before puberty. Before that age symptoms suggestive of this diagnosis will usually disappear with rest in a cylinder cast for three weeks. They may be caused by a partially torn tibial collateral ligament, or a contused cartilage or fat pad with persistent flexion deformity. In the adolescent, operation may be required. A torn cartilage or a discoid cartilage should be removed.

Fractures into Adjacent Epiphyses

Incomplete fractures of the upper tibial or lower femoral epiphyses are frequently referred to as knee injuries. Those of the lower femur have been discussed with fractures of that bone. More frequent in young children are the fractures into the proximal tibial epiphysis. A metaphyseal fracture without displacement may seem insignificant at first, but later may prove to be a serious injury of the growing cells of the epiphyseal plate resulting in valgus, varus, flexion, or back knee deformity. The prognosis must be guarded (Figs. 1, 2, pp. 4, 5 and Fig. 147, p. 106).

It must be remembered that angular deformity following fracture of the proximal end of the tibia may be the result of stimulation of one-half of the epiphyseal plate rather than retardation of the growth of the other. Roentgenographic measurement by six foot plates, scanograms, or by other accurate means should determine the length of the bone immediately after healing of the fracture. This record is invaluable in determining whether the subsequent deformity is due to overgrowth or retardation. The most frequent cause of growth arrest is the slightly displaced epiphyseal fracture with a crush injury of the metaphyseal plate due to a forceful longitudinal thrust, rather than the widely displaced epiphyseal fracture due to laterally directed trauma. In the latter case, the growing cells of the epiphysis are all carried with the epiphyseal plate. They continue to grow with temporary acceleration so that the shaft soon lines up with the displaced epiphysis. In the crush type of injury some of the cells are destroyed and growth is retarded thereafter.

Tibia vara (107) is a relatively common lesion of idiopathic origin. The infantile type is an exaggeration of the physiologic development. It may be unilateral (Fig. 233) or bilateral. The differential diagnosis from the preceding post traumatic lesion is easily made by roentgenograms. If a fracture occurs in a bone which was previously bowed, the diagnosis should be made at the time of the fracture. Frequently the original deformity may be corrected during the treatment of the fracture. The tendency to recurrence must be noted. Checkup roentgenograms should establish the accuracy of the alignment at the end of the healing period. If a varus (bow leg) develops later as a result of epiphyseal damage, the surgeon will then have proof that the reduction was accurate.

Tibia valga (Fig. 234), *femora vara*, and *femora valga* (107) are rare but have been observed as idiopathic lesions. Such deformities are usually due to injury or disease.

Before any angular or rotational deformity in the young child is ascribed to trauma or disease, the physician should be familiar with the normal variations of the developing child (108, 109, 110, 111). The newborn baby has flexed knees and hips. The knees are rotated externally while the feet are rotated inward. There is lateral bowing of both femora and tibiae. These "physiologic" deformities are normally overcorrected during the first two years of life. A three year old child has a knock knee-back knee stance with the feet pointing straight forward. A pre-adolescent girl should be appreciably knock kneed if the tibiae are to be parallel after the enlargement of the pelvis has occurred at puberty. If these "deformities" are corrected during the course of fracture treatment they will go on to overcorrection as the child develops.

DISLOCATIONS OF THE KNEE

Dislocation of one or both knees is occasionally observed at birth. The condition may be aggravated by the delivery, but is usually the result of a developmental anomaly with hyperextension and markedly restricted flexion. Treatment should be started promptly. With maintenance of the flexed position, it is sometimes possible to correct the deformity by conservative means. In the severe case, operation is indicated (126).

Traumatic dislocation of the knee is extremely rare in a child. It may be produced by great violence such as the impact of an automobile. Closed reduction and the application of a plaster cast will give a good result more frequently than in an adult. Forceful medial or lateral angulation of the knee in the adolescent may cause the complete avulsion of either end of the tibial or fibular collateral ligament. Novocaine injection of the tender ligament and roentgenograms taken with the knee in varus and valgus strain may be of great benefit in establishing the diagnosis. The knee joint will open widely under strain if the ligament is ruptured. The results with six to eight weeks of immobilization are satisfactory for ordinary activities but may preclude the prompt return to vigorous athletics. The question as to the management of such lesions will arise in the football injuries of high school boys. The operative replacement of the completely avulsed ligament should be considered if the case is diagnosed early. Recovery is more prompt and more complete. If the rupture is incomplete, or after a delay of a week, immobilization with a cylinder cast in extension and bowleg (or knock knee) strain, is the treatment of choice.

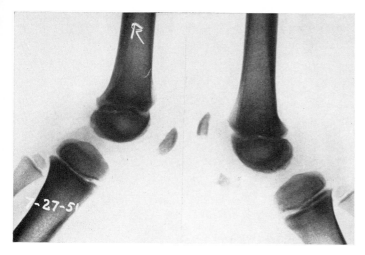

FIG. 221. D. J., male age 6, 7/27/51. A previous extensive laceration of the quadreicps mechanism limited flexion and predisposed to the transverse fracture of the left patella on sudden forceful flexion. This injury is rare in the child's normal knee.

FIG. 222. D. J., 8/13/51. The same case as in Figure 221, following repair of the extensor mechanism and approximation of the halves of the patella with stainless steel wire. Note that most of the patella is still cartilaginous. It looks as though the wire loop were too large. Recovery was complete with slight enlargement of the left patella.

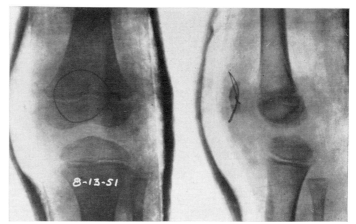

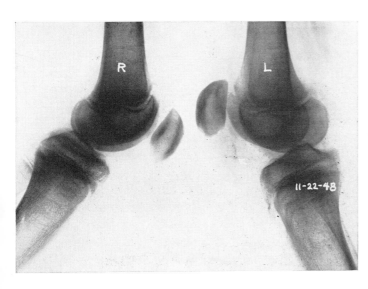

FIG. 223. H. Z., male, age 13. Sudden flexion of the left knee during a football game tore the extensor mechanism transversely. The patella was pulled upward and avulsed from the patellar ligament. The arrow points to the tiny chips of bone left on the ligament, indicating the former position of the patella.

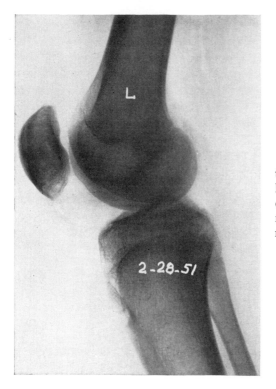

FIG. 224. H. Z., twenty-seven months following the preceding roentgenogram. There is complete healing after replacement of the patella in the distal ligamentous pocket and suture of the extensor mechanism. No internal fixation of the bone was necessary. An extension cast was worn for six weeks.

FIG. 225. J. M., male, age 16, with a history of a painful lump on the front of the right knee (Osgood-Schlatter's disease) of two years' duration. No adequate treatment. Note the separate ossicle which had formed in front of the patellar tubercle. This was a developmental anomaly and not a fracture. Separation had progressed too far for the lesion to heal by conservative measures. Excision of the entire area through a longitudinal incision in the patellar ligament resulted in a complete cure. Excision of only the ossicle does not relieve the symptoms.

Note the cortical cyst (non-ossifying fibroma) in the proximal end of the tibia. This is of no significance (see Chapter XVII, Pathologic Fractures).

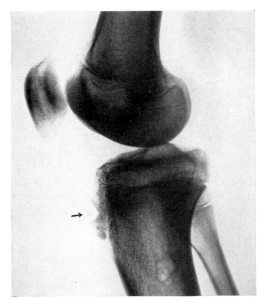

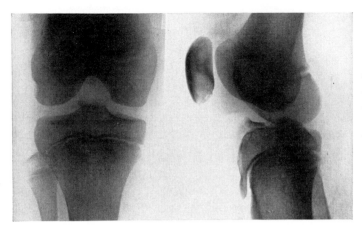

FIG. 226. E. B., male, 11/3/41. The portion of the tibial plateau to which the anterior cruciate ligament was attached was completely avulsed by the ligament. Symptoms of internal derangement were completely disabling. The knee could not be extended.

FIG. 227. E. B., 4/9/42, five months following the preceding roentgenogram. The avulsed fragment was replaced the day after the injury and maintained in position by a loop of stainless steel wire. Recovery of function was complete. The wire was easily removed.

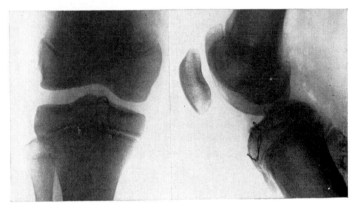

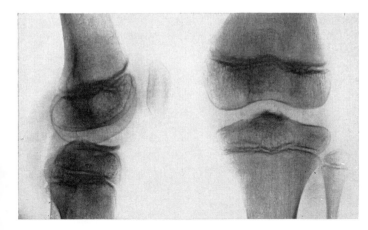

FIG. 228. S. V., female, age 8, 11/7/52. Avulsion of the anterior tibial cruciate attachment similar to that in the preceding case, but with less displacement of the fragment. Aspiration of the knee joint and immobilization of the knee with a long cylinder cast relieved the symptoms. (Courtesy of Dr. M. L. Straus.)

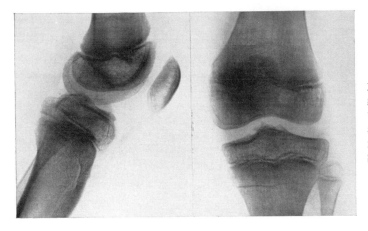

Fig. 229. S. V., 11/27/53. A year following the preceding roentgenogram shows complete healing with slight prominence of the avulsed fragment. Function was normal. (Courtesy of Dr. M. L. Straus.)

Fig. 230. W. K., male, age 15½, 1/23/39. The arrow points to a chip of bone and cartilage which was dislodged from the lateral femoral condyle when the patient jumped and twisted his knee in a basketball game.

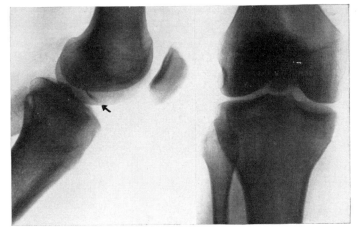

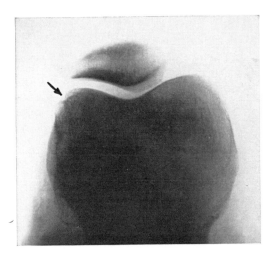

Fig. 231. W. K. A tangential roentgenogram of the preceding case showed the defect from which a chip of bone and cartilage was broken. Acute symptoms of internal derangement were produced. Removal of the free body was delayed for six months, and there was some residual disability with fibrillation of articular cartilage.

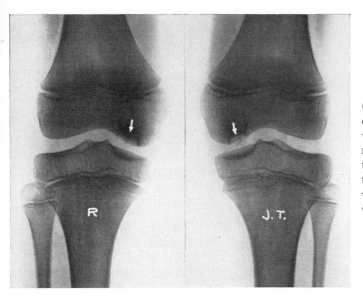

FIG. 232. J. T., female, age 10, 6/1/54. Bilateral osteochondrosis dissecans in an early stage. This was not a fracture. There had been no free body formation. Symptomatic treatment and immobilization of the knee with a cast for four to six weeks was all of the treatment that was necessary.

FIG. 233. Typical bilateral infantile type of tibia vara. The angular varus deformity was corrected by osteotomy near the proximal end of the tibia. Normal alignment was attained. This type is not as prone to recurrence as the adolescent. (Courtesy of Dr. Leo Mayer.)

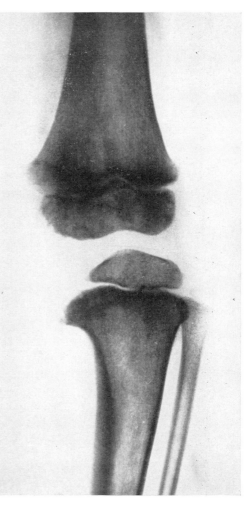

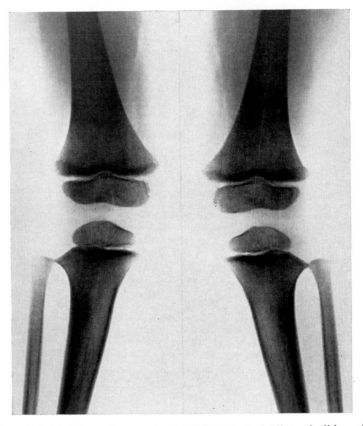

Fig. 234. M. H., male, age 3, 10/28/53. Typical bilateral tibia valga. This deformity and infantile tibia vara are developmental exaggerations of "physiologic" deformities. They are not produced by injuries of the epiphyseal plates. The deformity is rarely unilateral. (Courtesy of Dr. I. S. McReynolds.)

CHAPTER IX

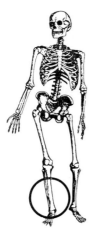

Injuries of the Leg and Ankle

THE SHAFTS OF THE TIBIA AND FIBULA

Fractures of the shaft of the tibia vary in character with the age of the child. In infants and children up to six years, torsion of the foot produces a spiral fracture of the tibia with no break of the fibula. There is frequently little or no displacement. This type of injury results from catching the foot in the crib and twisting in an effort to get loose. The older child falls with the foot caught and produces the same injury (Fig. 235). In children from five to ten years, direct trauma frequently produces a simple trans- verse fracture of both bones with or without displacement (Fig. 236). Among adolescents, sports such as skiing cause comminuted fractures of the middle third with butterfly fragments and marked displacement.

The *spiral fracture* of the infant frequently goes unrecognized. When the diagnosis is made the symptoms are relieved by a long leg cast from toes to mid-thigh, with the knee in flexion. This need be worn only three weeks. The similar fracture in an older child with minimal displacement needs immobilization for only four to five weeks in the same manner. When there is no fracture of the fibula, displacement sufficient to justify reduction is rare. Accelerated growth of the tibia corrects the slight bow ing. When *both bones* are broken and displaced, manipulation under anes- thesia will usually give satisfactory position. Bayonet apposition with 1 cm. of overriding is acceptable (Figs. 237–239 and Fig. 293, p. 244). A long cast with the knee bent is all the immobilization that is necessary (Fig. 240). When there is gross overriding with considerable displacement as in highway accidents, skeletal traction may be indicated, particularly if damage of the skin precludes the use of skin traction (Fig 256). A Kirschner wire may be inserted through the heel and the traction device incorporated in a cast extending to midthigh with the well padded knee slightly flexed (Fig. 240). Traction of five to ten pounds may then be placed on the cast and good alignment and satisfactory length maintained. As in the case of the femur, overriding of 1 cm. is considered a favorable position. Overgrowth in the leg occurs less rapidly but as consistently as it does in the femur (Fig. 257 and Fig. 294, p. 245). All closed leg fractures should be treated conservatively in children.

After the completion of growth, the complicated spiral ski or football fracture with a butterfly fragment and marked displacement, may require open reduction if an ideal end result is to be obtained. Closed reduction with overriding of the fragments, eventual slight shortening, and slight bony deformity are to be preferred to an attempted open operation by a tyro. Unless the injured youth is to have definitive surgery within an hour or two, before the swelling has become a problem, the leg should be immobilized in a splint or cast with a pressure dressing, ice bags, and elevation. It is unwise to attempt the open reduction of a tibial fracture at the height of the swelling a day after the injury occurs. It is better to wait several days until the reaction has subsided. Hyaluronidase may reduce this time. It should be emphasized that until growth is complete, open reduction has no place in the treatment of the fractured tibia. Even then, closed reduction and simple plaster fixation is usually the method of choice.

FRACTURES JUST ABOVE THE ANKLE

The typical ankle fractures of adults do not occur in children. Characteristic injuries occur for the various age groups. In the infant there is a *transverse greenstick fracture* just proximal to the epiphysis due to direct trauma (Fig. 236). The tibia alone, or both bones may be involved. There is usually minimal angulation, and immobilization with a long cast for three weeks is all that is necessary. In the child from three to twelve years, an ankle fracture often involves the epiphysis (Figs. 241, 244). As at the knee and wrist, the direct lateral force is less likely to produce growth arrest than the longitudinal thrust. The distal tibial epiphysis is the most prone of any in the body to the type of injury that causes damage to the epiphyseal plate and subsequent angular deformity and/or shortening (Figs. 242, 247).

Closed reduction of *epiphyseal fractures* at the ankle is usually easy if the case is seen promptly (Fig. 245). Open operation is not justified even with considerable residual displacement. A long cast with the knee flexed should be applied for four weeks in a young child. As puberty is approached the time should be extended to six weeks. It is imperative that the parents be informed that epiphyseal damage is not unlikely. Careful examination at intervals of three and then six months with accurate roentgenographic measurement of the individual bones is necessary for the first year or more until one can be sure that growth is progressing satisfactorily. Increase in length of the legs may be determined by direct measurement or by subtracting the sitting from the standing height. If there is no growth, an opinion as to progress must be deferred, even if considerable time has elapsed.

It is important to recognize an incipient deformity early so that the appropriate corrective measures can be instituted promptly before gross deformity has produced secondary changes (Fig. 243). A knowledge of the growth expectancy is important (Figs. 1, 2, pp. 4, 5 and 147 p. 106). When there is no epiphyseal damage, overgrowth of 1 cm. is the rule in a displaced fracture. This is equally true whether the fracture be in the middle of the bone or near the end.

Epiphyseal fractures with considerable displacement (Figs. 248, 249) should be treated with masterly neglect after a delay of two weeks. Closed reduction is usually impossible, and open operation is not justified. As previously discussed (Chapter VII) the growing cells accompany the epiphysis, and with molding, the angulation diminishes (Figs. 250, 251). As the child approaches puberty, more accurate reductions are necessary if unsightly deformity is to be avoided.

Malleolar fractures occur occasionally in older children with a version or rotational strain (Fig. 252). There is usually no displacement. On the lateral side, the epiphysis is likely to be involved. Here a fracture without displacement may go unrecognized until roentgenograms ten days later show subperiosteal callus about the epiphyseal plate. Malleolar fractures heal better than they do in adults. A short unpadded cast with a walking heel is usually the best treatment. Internal fixation is not necessary. Pseudarthrosis is not encountered in children.

SPRAINS

The feet of a normal child are pronated until the age of six years or more so that his ankles are extremely stable. Sprain is very rare. Foot strain is common. Overactivity and insufficient rest frequently cause ligamentous strain of the inner sides of the foot and ankle. A child with such strain often stands on the outer border of one or both feet with the toes curled under. He limps. He has a great urge to remove his shoes. Adhesive strapping with the heels inverted is a therapeutic test and good treatment.

An inside heel wedge with an elevation of $3/16''$ is good for the pronated foot of the older child. It should never be used on an infant who still walks on a wide base to maintain balance. Wedging the heels of the toddler will make his feet more unstable and prolong his awkwardness. Rigid arch supports have no place in the treatment of the feet of small children. Much of the thunder would be stolen from the shoe quacks who prey on over solicitous mothers if all doctors would broadcast the fact that small children are normally flat footed.

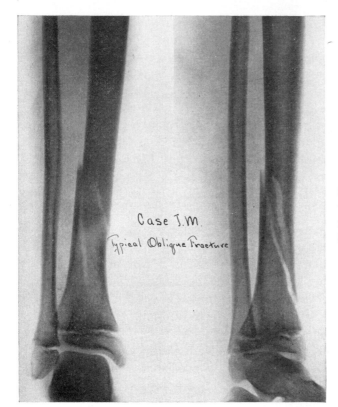

Case J.M.

Typical Oblique Fracture

FIG. 235. J. M., male, age 9. Spiral fracture of the distal third of the right tibia due to torsion. The fibula was not broken (other plates showed the proximal end).

FIG. 236. R. D., male, age 6. Typical greenstick fracture both bones of the distal third of the leg. Immobilization without reduction for five to six weeks in a long cast with knee bent.

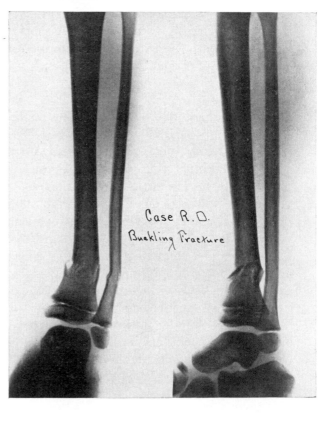

Case R.D.

Buckling Fracture

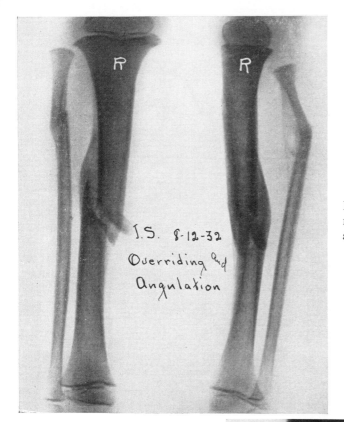

FIG. 237. J. S., male, age 4. Roentgenographic appearance on removal of the cast seven weeks after the fracture.

FIG. 238. J. S., seven years after the preceding roentgenogram. Function was completely normal.

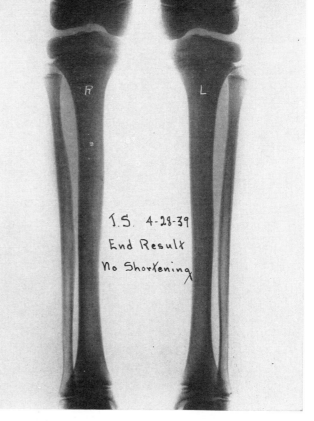

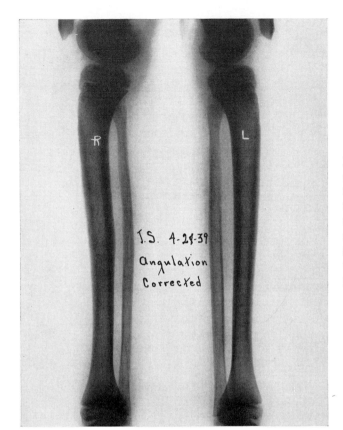

FIG. 239. J. S., lateral view to accompany Figure 238. The legs were roentgenologically symmetrical although the site of the fracture could still be identified. Moral: Bayonet apposition is acceptable. Moderate angulation of the middle of the tibia with the apex posteriorly is not productive of permanent deformity.

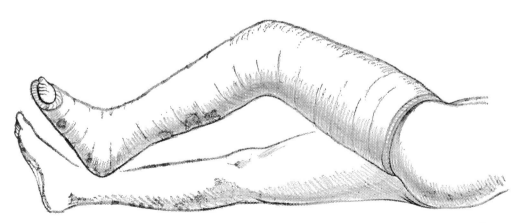

FIG. 240. Most fractures of the leg in children are well treated with a long leg cast. The foot should be at right angles and in neutral version. The knee should be flexed between 90° and 130°.

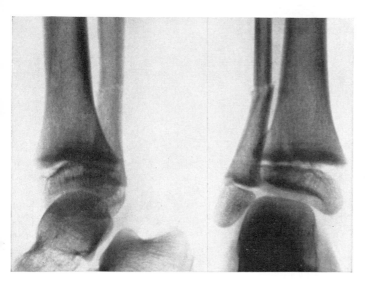

Fig. 241. C. M., female, age 6, 10/19/46. Fracture of the distal tibial epiphysis with greenstick fracture of the fibula healed satisfactorily without reduction. [Reproduced with permission of the American Academy of Orthopaedic Surgeons, Instructional Course Lectures (35).] (Courtesy, Dr. James J. Callahan.)

Fig. 242. C. M., 5/25/49, two years and seven months after Figure 241. There had been partial arrest of epiphyseal growth of the distal end of the tibia on the medial side. This had resulted in disabling varus of the ankle and shortening of the right tibia. [Reproduced with permission of the American Academy of Orthopaedic Surgeons, Instructional Course Lectures (35).]

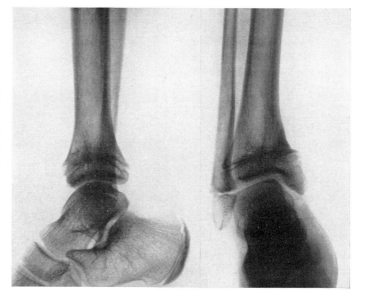

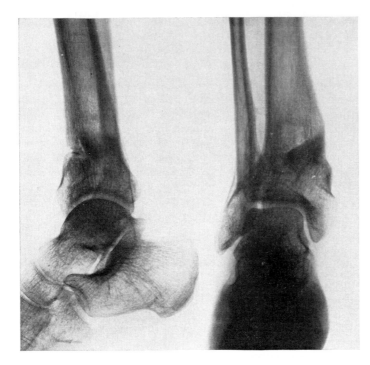

FIG. 243. C. M., 2/25/52. Three months after the second osteotomy to correct the angular deformity. A wedge shaped segment of cylindrical bone from the bank was inserted. There was complete correction of the deformity and good acceptance of the graft. This osteotomy will be permanent because there was epiphyseal closure. Inequality of leg length was equalized by stapling the proximal epiphysis of the opposite tibia. [Reproduced with permission of the American Academy of Orthopaedic Surgeons, Instructional Course Lectures (35).]

FIG. 244. E. E., male, age 8, 10/9/34. Distal tibial epiphyseal separation with oblique fracture of the middle of the fibula when the leg was crushed by an automobile. The view on the left is an oblique anteroposterior view, the right a lateral. [Reproduced with permission of the American Academy of Orthopaedic Surgeons, Instructional Course Lectures (142).]

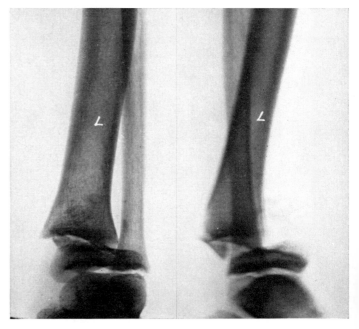

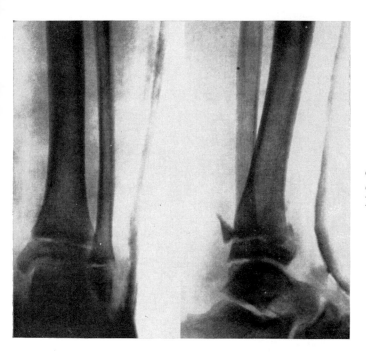

FIG. 245. E. E., 10/15/34. The preceding fracture after easy closed reduction and immobilization in a long leg cast.

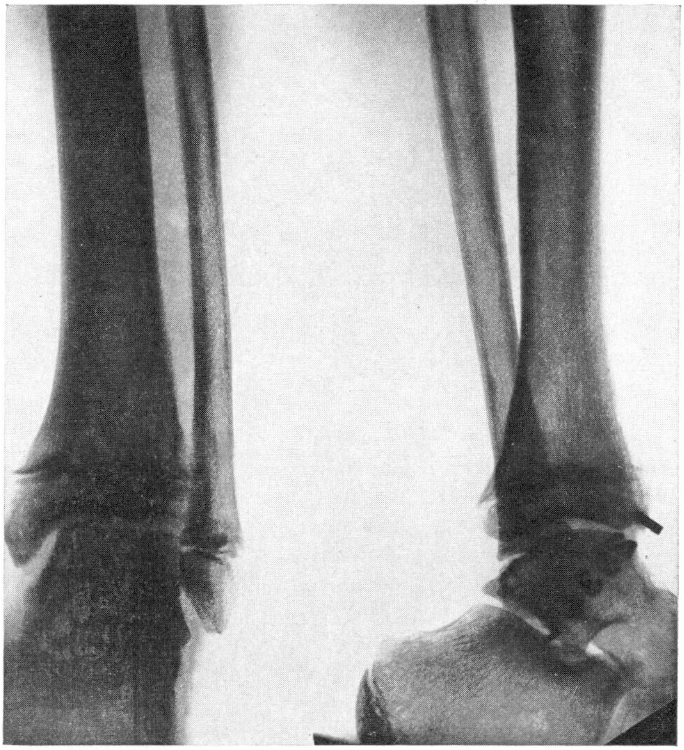

FIG. 246. E. E., 11/16/36. Two years after the fracture there was shortening of ½″ (12 mm.) due to injury of the distal tibial epiphyseal plate with slight varus of the ankle. [Reproduced with permission of the American Academy of Orthopaedic Surgeons, Instructional Course Lectures (142).]

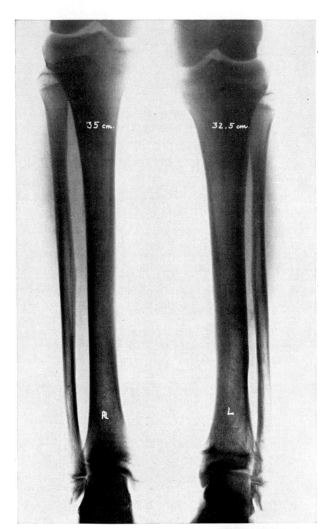

FIG. 247. E. E., 2/28/39, five years following the fracture shown in Figure 244. Epiphyseal growth was almost complete. There had been premature closure of the left distal tibial epiphysis. The varus deformity was minimal but there was 2.5 cm. shortening. Today we would anticipate the result at the end of the first two years and staple the opposite proximal tibial epiphysis. [Reproduced with permission of the American Academy of Orthopaedic Surgeons, Instructional Course Lectures (142).]

FIG. 248. B. P., female, age 10. Anteroposterior views of both ankles three weeks after a fracture on the right. There was 5 mms. of shortening. Moderate swelling. No treatment. [Reproduced with permission of the American Academy of Orthopaedic Surgeons, Instructional Course Lectures (35).]

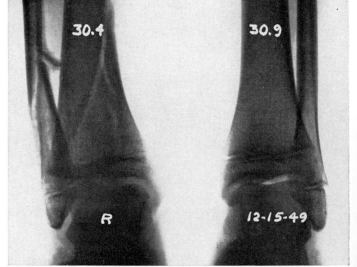

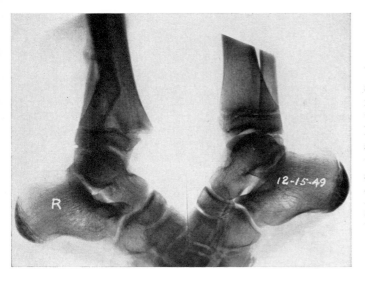

FIG. 249. B. P. Lateral views of both ankles of the preceding case show the deformity which was masked by swelling. The patient walked with crutches. Because of the likelihood of epiphyseal damage with attempted reduction, the deformity was accepted and a walking cast applied. [Reproduced with permission of the American Academy of Orthopaedic Surgeons, Instructional Course Lectures (35).]

FIG. 250. B. P. Anteroposterior view of both legs two years and four months following the preceding roentgenogram. The angular deformity was still visible but diminished and masked fairly well by the soft tissues. The right leg was now slightly longer than the left. [Reproduced with permission of the American Academy of Orthopaedic Surgeons, Instructional Course Lectures (35).]

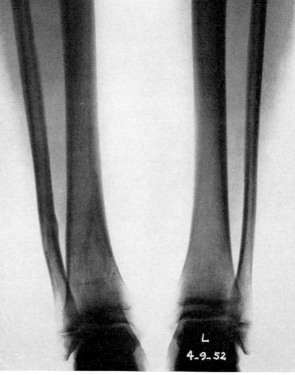

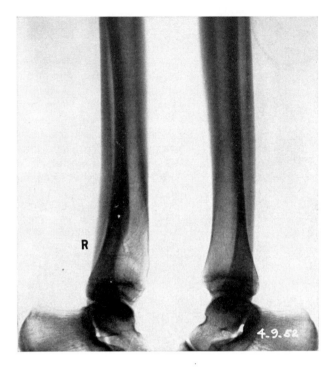

FIG. 251. B. P. Improved appearance in the lateral view as compared with Figure 249. The deformity was not clinically evident from the side. Note that the deformity in the saggital plane corrects better than deformity in the frontal plane. Moral: It is better to accept slight permanent angular deformity than run the risk of injury to an epiphyseal plate. [Reproduced with permission of the American Academy of Orthopaedic Surgeons, Instructional Course Lectures (35).]

FIG. 252. L. R., male, age 12. A longitudinal fracture through the medial side of the epiphyseal plate and metaphysis was immobilized in plaster without reduction. The fracture healed promptly and there was no growth disturbance.

CHAPTER X

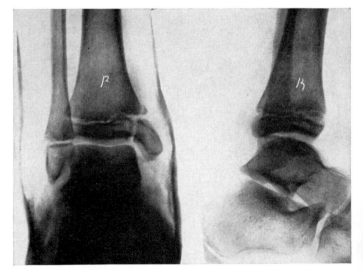

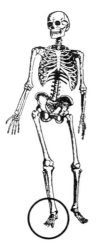

Injuries of the Foot[4]

The child's foot is so flexible and resilient that a force applied to it is usually transmitted higher up to produce the fracture there. Almost all fractures of the foot are due to direct trauma. A fall from a great height will cause a fracture of the calcaneus and/or the talus (Fig. 253) as in the adult, but lesser falls will break only the tibia. Crush injuries will fracture the metatarsals or the toes. Occasionally a child will stub his toe and break it, but not so frequently as his parents. Marching (fatigue) fractures which occur frequently in the metatarsals of adults are rare in children. Girls who skip rope vigorously in the spring after a long winter of relative idleness may develop a fatigue fracture of the second or third metatarsal. Callus may appear before the fracture line is visible. An osseous center at the base of the fifth metatarsal is normal until seventeen, and should not be confused with a fracture.

The recuperative power of the child's foot is tremendous. Except when the fracture is open (compound), operation is almost never indicated. A badly crushed foot (Chapter XVI, Open Fractures), is molded back to its normal contours and held in a padded plaster cast. The foot is elevated and surrounded by ice bags. The first cast soon becomes loose and is changed for an unpadded one. Metatarsals which look like a pile of jack straws will reshape themselves and with molding present a nearly normal roentgenographic apperance within a year or two. Function will be excellent. Angulated, closed metatarsal fractures are well treated with temporary skin traction on the toes and forefoot to produce better alignment. Skeletal traction on the phalanges is permissible but rarely necessary. Care should be taken to mold the arch. Broken phalanges should be splinted temporarily or bound to an adjacent toe. Good general alignment may be judged by the external contour of the toes.

Fractures of the talus, in contrast to those of adults (Figs. 254, 255),

[4] For "flatfoot" see the last two paragraphs, preceding chapter.

heal satisfactorily without serious residuals from avascular necrosis of the trochlea. Reasonably good position is necessary. The occasional displaced fracture of the talus with complete rotation of one fragment in an older child may require surgery to replace the fragment.

Flake fractures of the articular surface of the trochlea (Fig. 258) appear suddenly after a violent twist of the ankle of an older child (112) They may be difficult to demonstrate by roentgenogram unless the ankle is sharply plantarflexed. If displaced, they will not unite and must be removed like the chip fractures in the knee. The prognosis is good for normal function

The rare *fracture of the calcaneus* in a child should be treated conservatively. Amazing degrees of restoration of form and function have been observed. Mutilating operations are contraindicated. Avascular necrosis occurs, but creeping substitution is rapid (Fig 255). The subtalar post traumatic arthrosis which is so disabling in adults does not occur. The bone should be protected from weight bearing until it is revascularized.

Crush *fractures of the navicular* are almost unknown. Following an injury, the osteochondral lesion of this bone known as *Koehler's disease* (Fig. 259) (and a similar lesion of the cuneiforms) should not be confused with a fracture. The extreme flattening, fragmentation, and increased density of the osseous center are characteristic. Koehler's disease is self limited. Symptomatic treatment with a cast is desirable for three to four weeks until the tenderness and swelling have disappeared. After several months the roentgenogram will appear almost normal. Slight permanent thinning of the navicular is compatible with perfect function. There is no likelihood of permanent deformity as there is with coxa plana (Legg-Calvé-Perthes' disease).

Freiberg's disease (127) (Koehler's disease ⚹ 2) is a similar osteochondral lesion of a metatarsal head, usually the second or third, in a girl of about thirteen (Fig. 260). The entity is much more prevalent since the advent of loafers which cause pressure on the ends of the toes Pain frequently brings the patient in for roentgenologic examination There may be an osteochondrosis dissecans which is sometimes misdiagnosed as a fracture.

In contrast to Koehler's ⚹ 1, the prognosis is not good. Unless the disorder is recognized very early deformity results Weight bearing should be relieved by a cast in the severe case, or by appropriate modification with anterior pad and Jones' bar of a shoe that is long enough. Permanent limitation of motion is likely and the joint may become very painful in later life even requiring resection of the basal phalanx. The prevalence of this disease should constitute a plea for long enough shoes for growing girls.

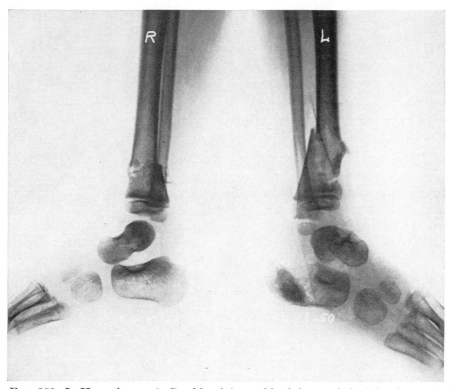

FIG. 253. L. K., male, age 3. Crushing injury of both legs and the left talus and calcaneus in a fall of five stories. After shock had been controlled, the legs were immobilized
in plaster using a Kirschner wire through the proximal end of the left tibia. There were also
fractures of the left femur, both ischial tuberosities, the sacrum, and several dorsal vertebrae. [Reproduced with permission of the American Academy of Orthopaedic Surgeons,
Instructional Course Lectures (35).]

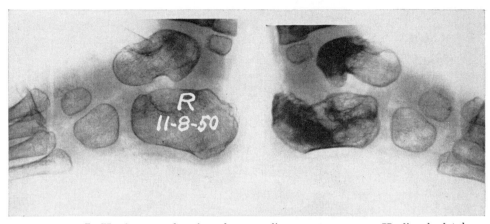

Fig. 254. L. K., five months after the preceding roentgenogram. Healing had taken place but there was avascular necrosis of the trochlea of the talus and the tuberosity of the calcaneus. [Reproduced with permission of the American Academy of Orthopaedic Surgeons, Instructional Course Lectures (35).]

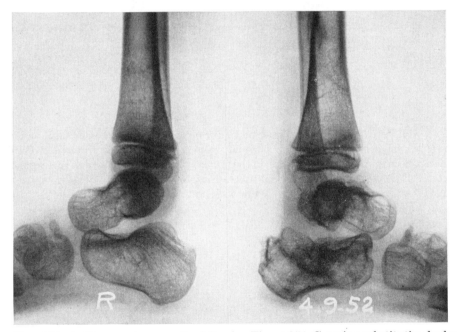

Fig. 255. L. K., seventeen months following Figure 254. Creeping substitution had occurred in the areas of avascular necrosis. Function was good although there was limitation of motion of the left ankle and subtalar joints. [Reproduced with permission of the American Academy of Orthopaedic Surgeons, Instructional Course Lectures (35).]

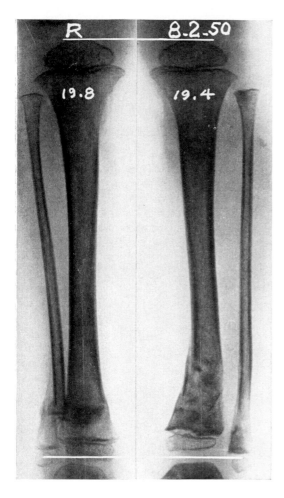

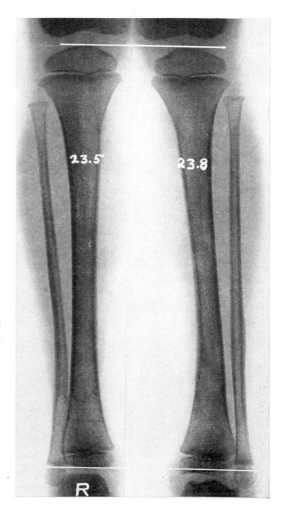

FIG. 256. L. K., a plate six weeks after Figure 253. There was 4 mm. shortening on the left. Note the channel of the Kirschner wire in the proximal end of the left tibia.

FIG. 257. L. K., 5/7/52. Two years following the preceding roentgenogram there had been a gain in the length of the left tibia of 7 mm. due to accelerated growth. The left tibia was now 3 mm. too long. Angular deformity was still visible but not disabling.

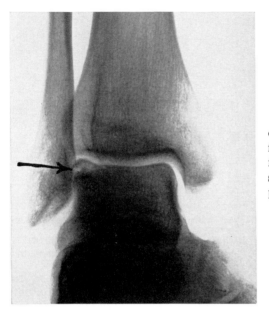

FIG. 258. M. E., female, age 13. A flake fracture of the trochlea of the astragalus was easily recognized five months after injury. In the original film the fracture was missed although it was visible on careful scrutiny. The ankle was treated as a sprain. Complete recovery after removal of the loose fragment.

FIG. 259. B. B., female age 4. Koehler's disease of the tarsal navicular; not a fracture. There was increased density, flattening, and fragmentation of the osseous center associated with swelling and pain. The symptoms were relieved by a walking plaster cast. The form of the navicular was gradually restored. The disease is self-limited. Significant deformity does not occur even without treatment.

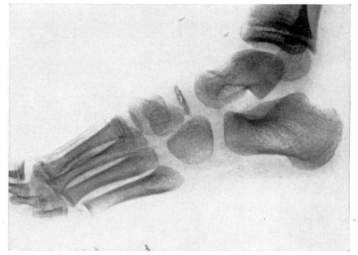

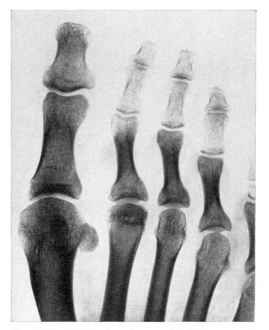

Fig. 260. P. W., female, age 14. This was not a fracture of the head of the second metatarsal. Freiberg's disease (Koehler's disease ≠2) is an osteochondral lesion similar to coxa plana. There is the same tendency to deformity if the foot is not protected at an early stage. Short shoes predispose to this lesion.

CHAPTER XI

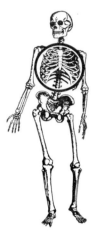

Injuries of the Ribs and Sternum

Like the fibulae, the *ribs* in children are so elastic that they are rarely broken except by a crushing injury. The general condition of the child is then the first concern and the fractures may be disregarded. Rib fractures in children due to a blow are likely to be greenstick. A swath made of an elastic bandage is comforting. A strip of muslin over one shoulder will keep it from slipping down (Fig. 261). A "Sam Brown belt" may be used. Adhesive produces more discomfort than the fracture in most cases.

Fractures of the sternum are of rare occurrence in older children. If the fracture is displaced, there is no trouble with closed reduction if treatment is prompt. The patient is placed in hyperextension with the arms above the head. Under local or general anesthesia the fracture is reduced by head and foot traction and digital pressure. In an old fracture, closed reduction is impossible. There is no indication for open reduction. Function is normal. Molding corrects any deformity.

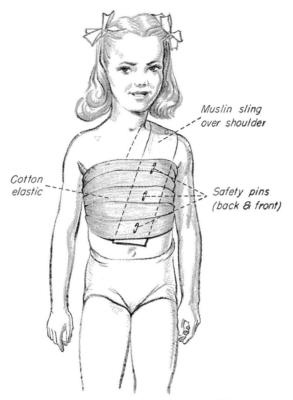

FIG. 261. Fractures of the ribs in children may be made more comfortable by a cotton elastic swath. It is kept from slipping down by a muslin band over the shoulder.

CHAPTER XII

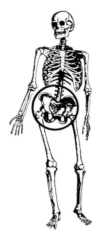

Injuries of the Pelvis

Crush fractures of the pelvis occur rarely in children of any age because of the elasticity of this bony ring with its interposed cartilage buffers. Unless they are complicated by injury of the urethra or other pelvic contents, they are of little significance. They heal very rapidly. Moderate degrees of malposition are of no significance as they disappear with molding. In older girls, restoration of the pelvic outlet is necessary. This should not require surgery. If the fragments are separated, they may be pulled together by a hammock (Fib. 262A). More commonly, there is compression of the pelvis (113). This may be corrected by the application of two long leg casts with a fulcrum at the knees and a turnbuckle or Spanish windlass to pull the feet together (Fig. 262B). Either type of force may be combined with traction on one leg if there is upward riding of one-half of the pelvis (Fig. 262A).

Boys between twelve and nineteen, rarely girls of equal development, may have a *traumatic separation of the apophysis of the ischium*. The crescent of bone is pulled away by a violent muscle effort such as a jump or a sudden start in running. When there is wide separation, union does not take place spontaneously and considerable disability results. There is weakness and pain with activity. When displacement is minimal, the apophysis will unite (114). Molding will correct the deformity if the adolescent grows for several years. Some thickening of the ischium persists when the injury occurs nearer the closure of the apophysis at the twenty-fifth year. Open operation and internal fixation have failed because of delay in some cases. The fragment has pulled loose again (115). An attempt at reduction and secure fixation of the grossly displaced fragment would be justified if the diagnosis were made early. Excision may be considered in the late case with disabling symptoms, but there is a marked tendency to the reformation of new bone at this location. The scar superficial to this bone is tender when the patient sits.

Just before the *ischiopubic hiatus* closes in children from four to eight years of age there is frequently a considerable exaggeration of the normal fusiform enlargement of the synchondrosis suggesting callus (Fig. 263). This osteochondral lesion (116) may cause a limp and limitation of abduction. It is not a fracture. A few day's rest is all the treatment that is necessary. The enlargement disappears with time.

Os acetabula may appear as a permanent separate ossicle at the rim of the acetabulum. The osseous center here may temporarily present the common picture of an osteochondral inflammatory lesion. Irregularity of ossification may give the appearance of a fracture (Fig. 264). The lesion is rarely symptomatic. If there is hip pain it will disappear spontaneously.

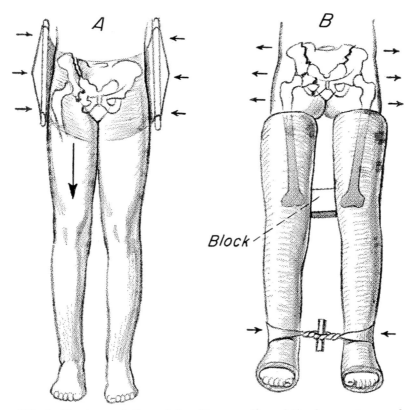

FIG. 262. A. Fractures of the pelvis with separation of the fragments may be controlled by a pelvic sling suspended by weights and pulleys on either side. If there is upward riding of the hip and ilium on one side, the sling may be combined with traction on the affected side as shown by the arrow. B. If the fragments are overlapped by compression, lateral separation of the femora is indicated. This may be obtained by applying long casts appropriately padded with felt in the groins, medial sides of the knees, and lateral sides of the ankles. A block is placed between the knees and the feet are approximated with a Spanish windlass. When the desired position has been verified by roentgenogram, the casts may be joined by plaster. Direct skeletal traction on the trochanters is impractical in children and likely to cause epiphyseal damage.

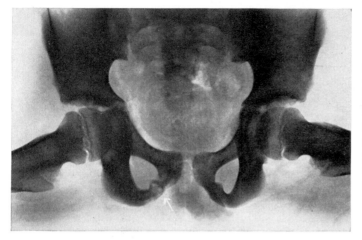

FIG. 263. J. D. Osteochondrosis of the ischial pubic hiatus is a lesion producing enlargement and irregularity of density. Symptoms of limp, usually without pain; limited abduction of the affected hip with other motions normal, are relieved promptly by bed rest. The roentgenographic changes may occur in the absence of symptoms.

FIG. 264. L. D. Irregularity in the development of the rim of the acetabulum may simulate a fracture in the roentgenogram. Symptoms of hip disability are rare. The center usually unites later, but may form an os acetabula. This was not a fracture but a bilateral osteochondral lesion associated in this case with abnormal development of the capital epiphysis.

CHAPTER XIII

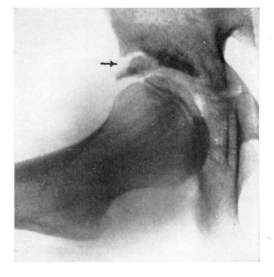

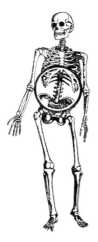

Injuries of the Spine

THE CERVICAL SPINE

Except in cases of extreme violence, *fractures and dislocations of the cervical spine* are rare. They occur in older children as diving accidents; rarely from the whiplash transportation injuries which are so common in adults. They are less likely to cause transection of the cord than are similar injuries of adults, but their treatment is otherwise essentially the same (117, 118). Following injury, an asymmetrical attitude may lead one to misdiagnose a congenital anomaly as a fracture. Roentgenograms should be carefully studied and compared with those of a child of similar age. Apophyses are often confusing. *Klippel-Feil syndrome*, failure of differentiation of the cervical vertebrae must be recognized as a congenital deformity.

Subluxation of a pair of facets of the cervical spine is relatively common; *complete unilateral dislocation*, more rare (Fig. 267). During a game a child's head may be jerked to one side and rotated. It remains in that position (Fig. 266) due to a failure of one pair of facets to return to the normal position. A subluxation is difficult to demonstrate on a roentgenogram but a complete luxation may be identified (Fig. 267). With head traction the pain and spasm will disappear and the involved facets will reseat themselves (Fig. 268).

A few days in bed with a pull of a felt harness (Fig. 268B) is usually the treatment of choice. The commercial Sayre head pieces are less comfortable. When neck motions are normally free and painless, a collar made of stockinet filled with coarse cotton is applied as illustrated (Fig. 269). It is more comfortable as well as more efficient than the adjustable neck braces sold by instrument houses and brace makers. It lifts the head with a definite traction effect. In older children a Minerva jacket (Fig. 265) may be preferable.

An acute subluxation may be reduced by manipulation without anesthesia. While traction is applied and the child is completely relaxed in the position of deformity the head is given a sudden deft twist in the direction of increased deformity. This unlocks the facets and permits them to seat again. The head should then be similarly manipulated in the opposite direction. The manipulation must be painless. Motions will then be entirely normal while traction is maintained. It is well to continue to support the neck for several days with a cotton collar (Fig. 269). Traction is not necessary when the subluxation is seen promptly and completely reduced. If there is any delay, traction in bed is the only treatment to consider.

Spontaneous dislocation of the atlas and axis may occur as a complication of upper respiratory disease (119, 120). A careful history should distinguish this entity from the preceding one. Bed rest with traction is indicated, never manipulation. A plaster collar may be desirable for a few weeks after the patient is ambulatory.

THE DORSAL SPINE

Small children may be tied in knots without fracturing the dorsal spine. After the age of eight years, a jack knife injury in football, a blow from a falling object, a fall from a height, or a transportation accident will compress a vertebra (Fig. 270), but the fracture is rarely unstable. Usually the compression is not great and it is unnecessary to reduce the deformity. Until healing is complete the child should be placed in a hyperextension cast to prevent further collapse. Active treatment without support, which is so desirable in most spine fractures of adults, is not applicable in relatively irresponsible children.

After a few weeks the roentgenogram will show some irregularity of contour and bone density due to osteochondral changes of the secondary osseous centers. The vertebral body will slowly become homogeneous and there may even be partial restoration of form (Fig. 271) if extension has been well maintained by a cast or a brace. No disability results even though there is slight permanent wedging.

In the absence of extreme violence, a fracture of the dorsal spine is likely due to a pre-existing lesion. Eosinophilic granuloma is one cause for collapse (Chapter XVII). There are occasional cysts of the vertebral bodies which disappear following the fracture. If a pathologic fracture produces lateral wedging of a vertebra (Fig. 272) the resulting local angular deformity should be held overcorrected for many months to be sure that the deformity does not progress during a rapid growth spurt. Reversal of the unequal pressure on the compressed vertebra permits equalization of the deformity by overgrowth of the involved and adjacent vertebrae according to Hueter (121) and Volkmann (122) and demonstrated repeatedly by Risser.

One must not mistake for a fracture an idiopathic osteochondral lesion of the primary (Fig. 273), or secondary (Fig. 274) osseous centers of the spine. The first, known as *Calvé's disease*, (128) and orginally believed to be an idiopathic osteochondrosis like coxa plana, is a lesion of the primary osseous center of a vertebra. The body becomes dense, very flat, and broader than the contiguous ones (Fig. 273). The adjacent intervertebral spaces are increased rather than diminished. With bed rest, the height of the vertebra is almost restored, and the density returns to normal. It is recognized now, with better roentgenograms, that several lesions may cause this symptom complex. In some, the loss of height may be occasioned by a pathologic fracture as in eosinophilic granuloma (Chapter XVII, Pathologic Fractures).

Scheuermann (140) was the first to describe the irregular development of the *secondary osseous centers* of the spine causing juvenile round back. The etiology is unknown. The deformity is probably associated with metabolic dysfunction. It is strongly hereditary. Increase in the deformity may be minimized by prompt efficient splinting (Fig. 275). Rapidly progressive curves are best treated by correction in a Milwaukee brace and prompt fusion. There is an immediate cosmetic improvement with definite roentgenographic evidence of correction of the kyphos. If fusion is solid, the deformity does not relapse, although the grafted area will elongate with further growth of the spine.

THE LUMBAR SPINE

In the *lumbar region* where the disorder is less frequent, the differential diagnosis is more difficult (Fig. 276). The isolated irregularity of development of a single epiphysis (Fig. 277) is often confused with a fracture. Remember that fractures of the spine are almost unknown in children below the first lumbar segment. One must not overtreat an adolescent or an adult as a result of such a mistaken diagnosis. Not only are there likely to be far reaching medicolegal complications, but grave and wholly unnecessary neurosis may develop from an otherwise trivial injury.

Fractures of the laminae or pedicles are exceedingly rare, but must be looked for in cases of extreme violence to the torso in which there is an element of torsion (Fig. 278). Although the fracture may be unstable, reduction is not necessary. With rest, complete recovery is the rule, and in children there is no indication for spinal fusion. The support of a cast or a brace and later a corset, may be indicated.

In the older child, the differential diagnosis between *fracture of a transverse process* and an *ununited apophysis* must be determined by careful scrutiny of several roentgenographic films. Roentgenograms after several weeks may be necessary to be certain of the diagnosis. A fracture will heal in the interval; the anomaly will remain unchanged.

Congenital anomalies in the low lumbar region are likely to be mistaken for fractures. *Spondylolisthesis* with an isthmus defect and some forward slipping of the superior vertebrae is usually diagnosed for the first time when back pain appears spontaneously at age thirty; or younger, when the low back is subjected to unusual strain such as a tour of military service. Occasionally a spondylolisthesis will become symptomatic in childhood. Such a case was followed from nine years until twelve (Fig. 279). Disabling symptoms were not relieved by the prolonged use of a surgical corset. Complete relief of symptoms was obtained by fusion of the fourth and fifth segments to the sacrum (Fig. 280). In a ten year followup the young man reported participation in basketball and all ordinary sports without disability.

Spondylolysis, the isthmus defect without the slipping, is diagnosed in the oblique roentgenogram, occasionally better in the lateral. It must not be confused with fracture of the isthmus which is sometimes caused by great violence. Later roentgenograms will show healing of a traumatic bone lesion.

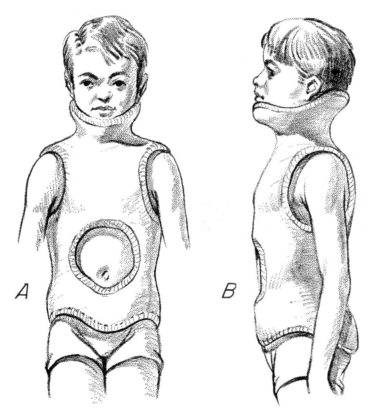

A   *B*

FIG. 265. Minerva jacket to be applied in the more serious injuries of the cervical and dorsal spine. It is useful in children who will squirm out of almost any neck brace that is known.

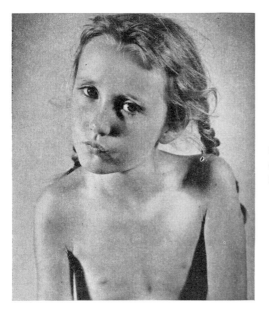

FIG. 266. M. M., female, age 6. A wry neck produced by a jerk on the head with painful subluxation of the facet between one and two on the right (Fig. 267).

FIG. 267. M.M. A. 8/13/52. Subluxation of the facet between the first and second cervical vertebrae on the right. B. 10/27/52. Head traction (Fig. 268) promptly reduced the subluxation. She wore a cotton collar (Fig. 269) for two weeks. Nine weeks after the injury the symptoms had completely disappeared.

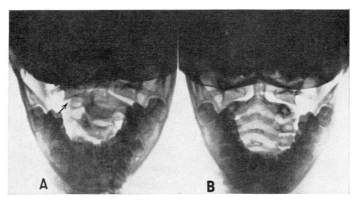

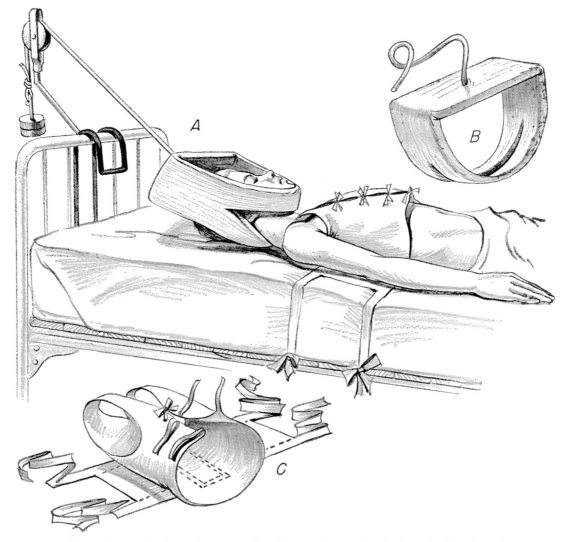

Fig. 268. A. Head traction with elevation of the head end of the bed is the safest method of treating neck injuries in children. B. A sling made of felt and stockinet is better tolerated than the commercial article. C. A restraint is necessary for most children.

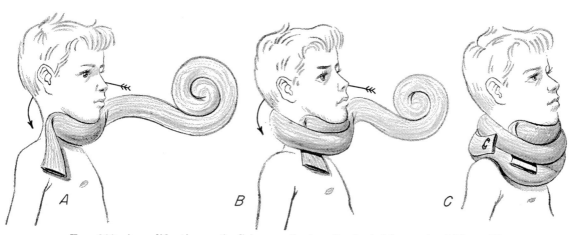

FIG. 269. A modification of the Schanz collar is well adapted for use in children. Three inch (17 cm.) stockinet six feet (2 m.) long is stuffed with coarse cotton. The cotton is first rolled lengthwise into a sausage and then pulled into the rolled up stockinet. Some empty stockinet is left at each end. The support is applied loosely under the chin and occiput (A). The second turn is below the first and somewhat tighter (B). The third turn is made snug enough to make the child uncomfortable at first. The first end is incorporated in the bandage and the loose end is pinned fast. This dressing may be tightened by the mother at frequent intervals. It affords a support to the head with a distraction effect on the neck.

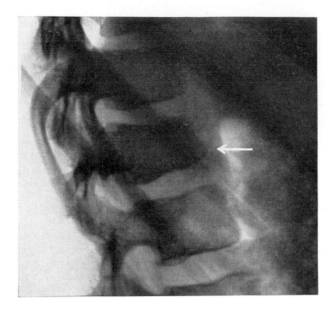

Fig. 270. T. O., male, age 11, 11/4/47. A compression fracture of the twelfth thoracic vertebra was sustained when this patient was "jack-knifed" while playing football with larger boys. Immediate pain in the back. There was compression of the superior table of the twelfth thoracic vertebra with an anterior break in the cortex. A hyperextension cast was applied for eight weeks followed by a hyperextension brace for a year.

Fig. 271. T. O., 11/28/52. Ossification was very irregular for several years in the compressed thoracic vertebra shown in Figure 270. After five years it had been partially reformed. There were no symptoms referable to the back. Clinical recovery was complete except for slight gibbus at the site of the fracture.

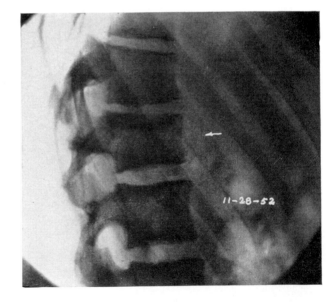

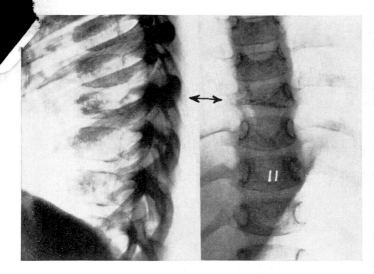

FIG. 272. K. V., female, age 6. Pain in the back associated with compression of the ninth thoracic vertebra immediately following a fall on level ground. The child landed on her back with her spine flexed. There may have been lateral flexion as well. Pain persisted until she was immobilized in a cast. For a year she wore a Milwaukee brace with a lateral strap on the left. Note the compression of the ninth thoracic vertebra on the right side. The fracture appeared to have occurred at the site of a preexisting cyst involving the right side of the body and right pedicle.

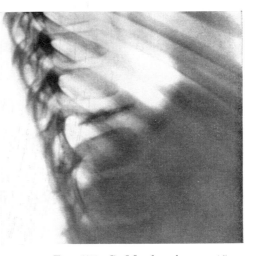

FIG. 273. F. M. This is one of the two cases published by Calvé (128). Collapse of a vertebra of a young child with broadening, increased density and sometimes fragmentation has since been identified with Calvé's name. Other cases have been cited in the literature with subsequent restoration of almost normal height and form. It is now recognized that several vertebral lesions of known etiology may cause this unusual sequence. (Courtesy of Dr. Elliott G. Brackett.) [Reproduced with permission of the Journal of Bone and Joint Surgery (128).]

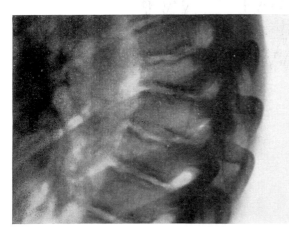

FIG. 274. G. M., female, age 15. An osteochondral lesion of the secondary osseous centers of the dorsal spine associated with ragged development of the vertebral epiphyses and anterior wedging of the involved vertebrae is associated with the name of Scheuermann (140). If the process is limited to one or two vertebrae it may be confused with fracture. Pain may be considerable while the disease is active. The permanent rounding of the back is objectionable particularly in girls. The disease is self-limited but may be greatly improved by maintaining proper posture during the active stage.

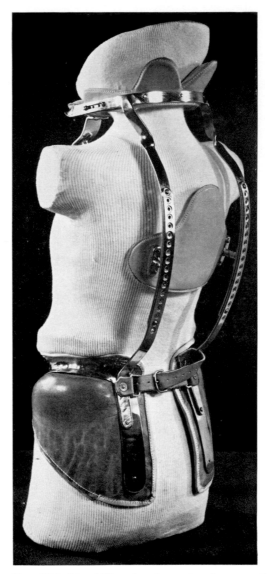

FIG. 275. The Milwaukee brace has been modified to treat vertebral epiphysitis (Figs. 274 and
276) in its active stage. It is used also following
spine fusion in the severe cases. It is equally adapt-
able to use in high dorsal fractures in children. In
the case in Figure 272 the brace was used with a
left lateral strap to correct the lateral deviation of
the spine.

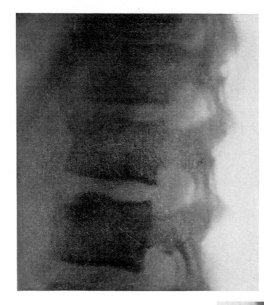

FIG. 276. I. S., female, age 12. Localized epiphysitis in the lumbar region is more likely to be confused with fracture. Pain was present in the active stage and the lumbar curve was reversed.

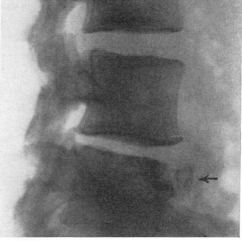

FIG. 277. Developmental anomaly of a lumbar vertebra. This is not a fracture. This lesion is sometimes the sequel to the vertebral epiphysitis seen in figure 276.

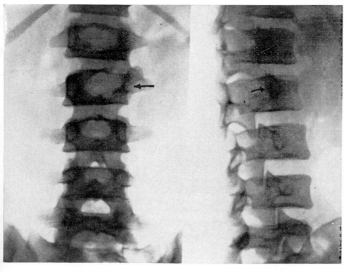

FIG. 278. M. K., female, age 5½. The lamina on the left side of the second lumbar vertebra was fractured when this child was struck in the back by a car. The anterior displaced articular facet is clearly visible in the oblique view (right). The lamina of lumbar one is tilted. The child was treated on a Bradford frame and made a comelete recovery clinically. There were no neurologic symptoms.

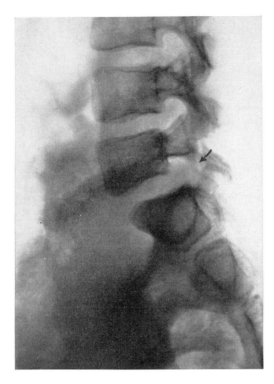

Fig. 279. A. E., male, age 11, 10/1/45. Spondylolisthesis caused disabling symptoms in spite of an efficient surgical corset. The defect in the pars intra-articularus which is visible in the lateral view (sometimes better shown in an oblique view) should not be confused with a fracture. It is usually developmental in origin. There is grade one forward slipping of the fifth lumbar vertebra on the sacrum. The fourth and fifth lumbar vertebrae were fused to the sacrum.

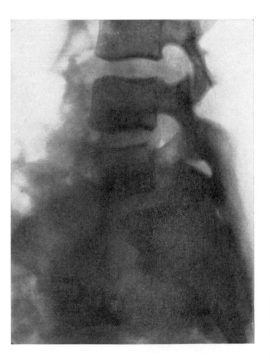

Fig. 280. A. E. Roentgenographic appearance one year after the operation in the case shown in Figure 279. The graft firmly united the fourth and fifth lumbar vertebrae to the sacrum. The symptoms were completely relieved.

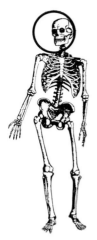

CHAPTER XIV

Facial Bone Fractures and Dislocations[5]

Etiology

Facial bone fractures in children are uncommon. Dislocations are limited to the temporomandibular joint and are even more rare. The potentialities for disfigurement and dysfunction are so great that immediate diagnosis and definitive treatment are necessary. Even with *good* treatment, disturbances in growth may be disfiguring in later years (123). The parents should be acquainted with this fact.

General Considerations

Open wounds with copious bleeding offer sufficient stimulus to the parent to bring the child to the physician for attention. Closed fractures may be promptly obscured by the rapidly appearing edema and swelling. If the parents rationalize that "everything is going to be all right and Johnny just had a bad bump", treatment may be postponed, or even omitted until too late for an optimum result. In closed injuries, the surgeon must suspect a fracture under an area of contusion and swelling. Diagnosis by gentle palpation must supplement mere inspection. Speculum examination is indicated in all nasal contusions. Palpation as well as observation of occlusion is necessary in injuries about the jaws. Examination of extraocular function must supplement palpation of the bony orbit in cheek injuries.

The most common injuries of the face are to the nose, mandible, maxilla, and malar bones in that order. They are most frequently caused by direct impact of the windshield or tonneau of a car, a hurtled object, or a

[5] This chapter was contributed by Dr. William H. Frackelton, Assistant Professor of Surgery, Marquette University, School of Medicine.

blow from the fist. A child's fall injures a nasal bone more frequently than the mandible, maxilla or malar bone.

Roentgenograms are essential for quantitative as well as the qualitative analysis of facial injuries. They may not reveal some nose injuries, but are essential in mandible, maxilla and malar bone fractures. Temporomandibular joint dislocations can be adequately diagnosed by palpation and testing dental occlusion, but should be verified by roentgenograms for the record and for an estimate of progress.

Treatment of closed fractures and dislocations can well be considered in conjunction with open injuries since manipulation and fixation proceed along similar methods.

Lacerations or avulsions require prompt attention and usually this is obtained. The repair should be exacting in order to prevent deformity. The rich vascularity allows primary closure of soft tissue wounds of the face eighteen or twenty-four hours after injury, much later than those of the extremities (Chapter XVI). This leeway should not be used as an excuse for undue delay. It does serve to provide sufficient time for roentgenograms, accurate diagnosis of fractures, treatment of shock, and evaluation of other injuries requiring simultaneous care.

It is unnecessary to postpone treatment of injury of the face because of coexisting cerebral damage. Even in children much can be done under local anesthesia if general anesthesia is temporarily contraindicated. With open face injuries, it is best to treat underlying fractures simultaneously rather than to follow the frequent practice of repairing lacerations and deferring treatment of fractures for several days. If fractures are treated early, reduction is easier, less traumatic, and less likely to cause growth disturbance. In addition, an open wound may give ready access to an underlying fracture and permit direct manipulation without accessory incision.

INJURIES OF THE NOSE

Palpation for abnormal movement and for crepitus is important. Intranasal inspection will reveal laceration of the mucosa, dislocation of nasal cartilage or septum, and the presence of hematoma requiring evacuation. Treatment is usually uncomplicated except for severe comminution involving the nasal bones as well as the septum. In the older child a preliminary barbiturate sedation and 5 per cent cocaine cotton intranasal packs supplemented with novocaine infiltration provide satisfactory anesthesia. In the younger child general anesthesia is needed for complete inspection as well as treatment.

Reduction is easily carried out by the use of a blunt instrument or a rubber sheathed probe in the nose, and finger manipulation externally.

Elevation and correction of lateral deviation will bring about realignment. The less comminuted fractures are relatively stable. The severely comminuted fractures require the supportive splinting of a light intranasal packing of fine mesh vaseline gauze in each nostril and up into the nose. This separates the septal from the lateral wall. A section of small rubber tube laid in the floor of each nostril serves, not so much to allow breathing, as to prevent discomfort during the act of swallowing with obstructed nostrils. The tubes are held from slipping back into the nasal cavity by an external suture passed through them and across the midline (Fig. 281). The suture in turn is held in place with a small piece of adhesive.

The nose is protected externally and stabilized further by a lightly padded metal splint. Light sheet aluminum or copper is best, but a splint can be cut from a tin can and bent into proper shape (Fig. 281). It is held on the nose with a central strip of adhesive fastened to the forehead. Adhesive strapping is applied transversely across the cheeks to keep the splint in contact with the nose and to prevent lateral displacement. The intranasal packing may be removed in two days if internal support is not needed. When internal support is required because of severe comminution of the septum, the packing may remain for as long as a week, but it is better to replace it before that time. The external splint should be maintained for ten to fourteen days to allow fibrous and bony union and also to prevent inadvertent trauma and displacement of the fractured nose.

Even minor injuries to the nose are likely to result in deformity. Well reduced nasal fractures may develop overgrown bony ridges requiring rhinoplastic correction in later years. The operation for improvement of the shape of external nose and septum is best postponed until the age of fifteen or sixteen. Occasionally severe septal thickening or displacement may require earlier attention (124).

MANDIBULAR FRACTURES

Mandibular fractures (125) are diagnosed by disturbances in occlusion. Light palpation will reveal the irregularity or tenderness of a fracture. Ecchymoses under the mucosa will point to the fracture site.

Early treatment is directed to maintenance of an airway. The child should be transported in the prone position with the face down and head lowered rather than supine. Bandages are frequently unnecessary except for lacerations. The commonly applied Barton bandage is actually harmful in that it forces the lower jaw backward and upward. A barrel type hitch (Fig. 282) is better and may be utilized even for definitive retention in some cases.

Left and right lateral roentgenograms show the vertical ramus of the mandible, the angle, and the body. Posteroanterior projections show the complete mandible. Specialized views or laminographic and stereoscopic films may be needed to visualize correctly the temporomandibular joint, the condyle, and coronoid process.

Uncomplicated fractures of the body of the mandible are adequately treated by manipulation, alignment in good occlusion, application of a barrel type hitch, and overlying plaster strips.

More severe fractures and those with marked displacement require reduction under anesthesia. Fixation by interdental loop wires at molar, canine, and incisor positions is suitable in the older child (Fig. 283). When only deciduous teeth are present, bands or wires are ineffective. Acrylic splints can be used. Extraoral fixation by pins is inadvisable for fear of damaging unerupted tooth follicles. A fracture at the angle of the jaw may require a small infra-angular incision and direct wiring through small bone drill holes even in children. The wire need not be removed. At the symphysis a similar method is feasible or a transfixion Kirschner wire may be placed in the lower portion of the symphysis without damage to tooth follicles. Accompanying condylar dislocations are corrected by bringing the teeth into occlusion. When necessary a thickness of rubber can be placed between the upper and lower teeth to act as a fulcrum during part of the period of gradual reduction and splinting.

Subcondylar fractures are treated similarly by reducing them and bringing the teeth into occlusion for fixation. The potentialities of growth disturbance are great since the greatest elongation of the mandible occurs in this area.

Following reduction and during retention of the jaw in occlusion, the young child can be fed with a rubber tube attached to a syringe. An ordinary diet run through a blender can be managed by the older child through available tooth spaces. It is unnecessary to extract a tooth.

A simple mouth wash should be used after each feeding.

An antibiotic should be given prophylactically in open fractures.

Much of the foregoing applies to fractures of the maxilla (125). When the alveolar process alone is involved, the loose teeth are supported on an arch bar stabilized to the adjacent teeth. In small children, acrylic splints may be necessary. Extensive maxillary fractures require specialized fixation.

Malar Fractures

Malar fractures may be limited to the zygomatic arch. A palpable depression may exist and there may be accompanying difficulty in jaw action due to coronoid impingement or involvement of temporal and masseter muscle. If the injury is limited to this area, elevation of the fracture can be carried out. The bone may be simply elevated by a hook introduced subcutaneously. More severely displaced arch fractures require a temporal incision and elevation of the arch by a probe passed beneath the temporal fascia. After reduction the fracture is stable unless it is severely comminuted.

INFRAORBITAL FRACTURES

When a malar fracture is confined to the orbital rim, the diagnosis is made by palpation. Abnormal extraocular movement should be noted. The cooperative older child should be tested for diplopia. Fracture in this area frequently involves the infraorbital foramen and infraorbital nerve and leads to numbness of the cheek, nose, and lip. If the nerve is severed, paresthesia and hypesthesia may be permanent.

Treatment of *infraorbital fracture with displacement* is suitably carried through an infraorbital incision, direct exposure of the bone, and elevation of the fracture by a hook. If the infraorbital floor is severely comminuted the antrum is entered through a buccal incision. The antrum is cleared of blood and torn mucous membrane and packed sufficiently firmly with vaseline gauze strips to elevate the orbital floor and correct any ocular displacement. Instead of leading the pack out through the buccal incision within the junction of the gum and cheek, a nasal aperture can be made with a blunt hemostat and the pack led out through the nose. The buccal intraoral incision can then be closed with less opportunity for an oral-antral fistula to form. The pack remains in place for two weeks and it is then withdrawn in stages.

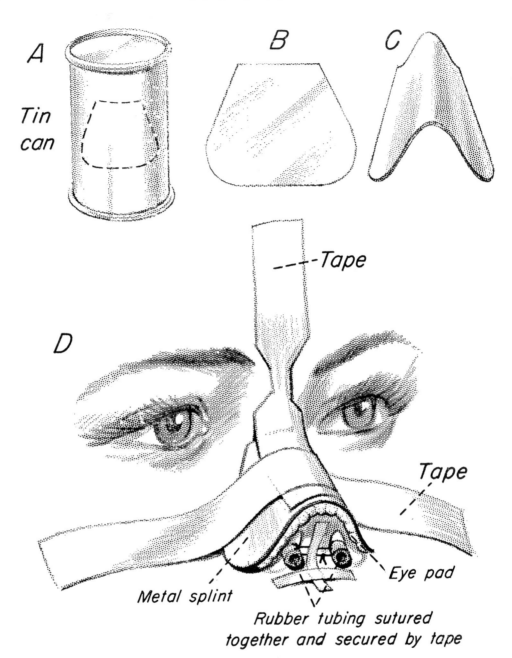

A

*Tin
can*

B

C

D

- - - -*Tape*

Tape

Eye pad

Metal splint

*Rubber tubing sutured
together and secured by tape*

Fig. 281. Splinting of an injured nose. A. and B. A light aluminum nasal splint is best. A can may be cut with tin snips according to pattern shown, as an effective substitute. C. The splint is bent to the shape of the nose. D. After reduction and suture of the injured parts, the position is maintained by intranasal petrolatum gauze packing. Within the gauze packing but along the floor of the nose 2½ inch (6 cm.) rubber tubes will provide an air channel. The skin of the nose is painted with tincture of benzoin, overlaid with transverse strips of adhesive, and the metal splint applied. If there are external lacerations, a thin fine mesh gauze padding (eye pad) is used instead of adhesive tape. In children especially, it is necessary to prevent the displacement of the intranasal gauze packing and rubber tubes by an external stitch through the gauze and rubber from side to side as shown.

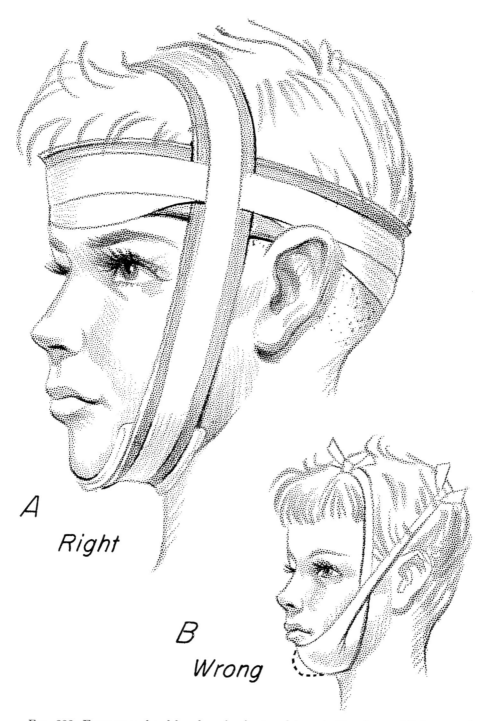

FIG. 282. Emergency head bandage for fractured jaw. A. Barrel type hitch supports without retracting the lower jaw. B. Barton type hitch incorrectly forces the lower jaw posteriorly and thus causes tongue obstruction of the airway.

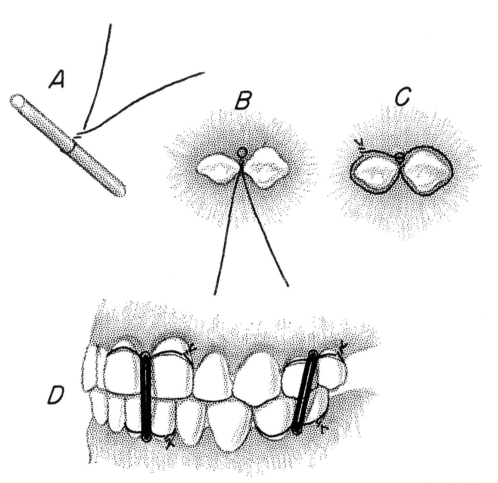

Fig. 283. Method of applying interdental fixation. A. A 6-inch (15 cm.) length of #28 or #26 wire (.012 cm. or .016 cm.) is given a single twist about a rod of $\frac{3}{32}$ inch (.23 cm.) diameter. B. Both ends of the wire are passed between the selected pair of teeth at the gum line. C. One end of the wire is brought about the crown of each tooth and one end is passed underneath the twisted loop before it is approximated to the other. The twisted loop is then given additional turns to make the fixation snug. D. After the paired wires are in place, small rubber bands (may be cut from a rubber tube) are placed over the twisted loops as shown.

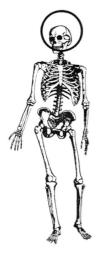

Skull Fracture and Craniocerebral Injuries[6]

ETIOLOGY

Injuries to the brains of infants during delivery are less common than was previously believed. There is often some underlying abnormality predisposing to cerebral injury during delivery. The actual cerebral defect usually exists prior to birth. The designation, "birth injured" is unfortunate and should be replaced by "cerebral palsy".

The incidence of skull fractures and craniocerebral injuries in children has increased in direct proportion to the gain in the number of vehicles and the speed at which they travel. The number of children injured in autos, by cars while at play or while crossing the street has grown to an alarming level. Falls from porches and windows have added to the toll. The spreading distribution and increasing number of these cases calls for understanding of the basic principles of treatment of head injuries by the general physician or surgeon. This requires knowledge of the fundamentals of anatomy and physiology of the nervous system.

GENERAL CONSIDERATIONS

The skull of the child must be considered in three stages of development. The first phase is that of the infant skull with open suture lines. In the second, the suture lines are joined but ossification is incomplete. In the third, the skull is completely ossified like a rigid box. The transmission of force through the skull to the brain varies with the phases of development. A blow on the inelastic closed box skull transmits the force in all directions through the semicolloidal brain and its fluid envelope. The presence of the foramen magnum, minor foramina, nerves and blood ves-

[6] This section was prepared by Dr. David Cleveland, Professor of Neurologic Surgery, Marquette University, School of Medicine.

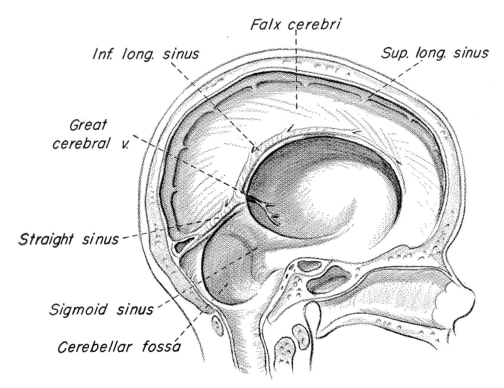

Fig. 284. Midsagittal section of the head

sels, dura, falx, and tentorium alters the mechanism only slightly (Fig. 284).

The skull with closed suture lines, but incomplete ossification is much more elastic than the rigid box. It will absorb some of the blow and lessen the force transmitted to the brain. The effect of trauma to the infant skull with patent sutures is more local with minimal transmission through the brain, because of the great elasticity of the unfused portion of the skull.

The lines of stress of the skull and the mechanism of skull fracture are well recognized. With impact, there is an area of inbending immediately beneath and around the point of the blow. Surrounding this is an area of outbending which has a tearing apart effect. If the force is adequate and the velocity high, the area of inbending fails and a depressed fracture results. If the area of inbending does not fail, the tearing apart effect may result in a linear fracture which radiates from the point of impact. The type of fracture depends upon the speed and energy of the blow. The high velocity injury tends to cause perforation and depression at the point of impact. A blow of low velocity and great force causes a stellate fracture with depression of an extensive area.

The elastic skull of the infant with meager ossification absorbs much of the blow by the give of the skull plate as a unit. A blunt object striking this membranous type of skull with low velocity will cause a "derby hat" deformity (Fig. 291); a dent in the elastic skull without tearing apart or fracture. The elastic inbending from a low velocity blow may dissipate the force and permit relatively little cerebral injury. High velocity force results in severe local cerebral injury due to ineffective skull protection.

The presence of a fracture in the skull is of minor importance, unless it crosses a sinus so as to admit air or infection into the cranial cavity, or tears a blood vessel or nerve. In contrast to fractures elsewhere in the body, there is no muscle pull to add deformity. The prime consideration is not that of the fracture, but rather of the brain damage.

When sudden force is applied to the skull, there is an immediate increase in intracranial pressure which can be measured. At the same time there is a sudden movement of the brain, which is most marked at the midline or falx. This is followed immediately by a rebound stretch. As a result of the brain movement and increased tension, there may be severe molecular and chemical alterations, small blood vessel rupture, and petechial hemorrhage throughout the brain. The rebound stretch may tear the surface vessels and cause subdural or extradural hemorrhage.

When the skull is moved by sudden force, there is a slight lag in the movement of the brain, due to its inertia in its fluid envelope. Conversely, when movement of the skull stops suddenly, the brain moves further. Lacerations and hemorrhages may occur in the frontal and temporal lobes from the trauma of the ridges of the floor of the skull.

The cerebrum consists of two hemispheres which are separated by a tough, sickle shaped falx which extends from the anterior tip to the tentorium behind (Fig. 284). The tentorium divides the cerebral hemispheres from the cerebellum which lies behind and below. The brain stem runs through an opening in the tentorium to the pons which is surrounded above and laterally by the cerebellar hemispheres. Severe disturbances frequently occur at this opening in the tentorium. Massive increase in pressure above the tentorium may force the uncal portions of the temporal lobe to herniate through the incisura and compress the brain stem to such a degree that its function is abolished. Decerebrate rigidity may result from such herniation.

The effects of cerebral injury depend to a great extent upon alterations of the arterial, venous, and cerebral spinal fluid circulation. The cerebrospinal fluid is produced largely by the choroid plexus lining the ventricles. It circulates from the lateral ventricles through the foramen of Monro into the third ventricle, and then by way of the aqueduct of Sylvius to the fourth ventricle in the posterior fossa. It escapes into the subarachnoid

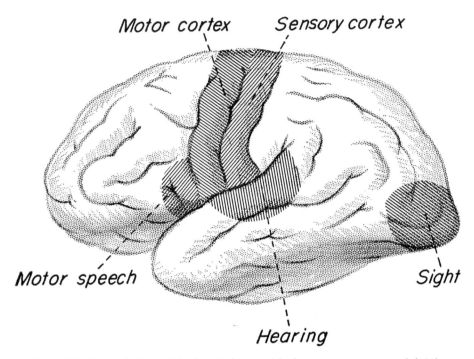

FIG. 285. Lateral view of the hemispheres with the motor areas named (129)

spaces by way of the two lateral foramina of Luschka, and into the cisterna magna through the medial foramen of Magendie. It leaves the cisterna magna between the inferior portions of the cerebellum, to enter the subarachnoid space around the cord and brain. The fluid is absorbed into the venous sinuses through the archnoidal villi and granulations to complete circulation. The flow is aided by the pumping effect of the arterial pulsations of the brain. Increase in the volume of the brain may compress the subarachnoid spaces and impair circulation and absorption of the cerebrospinal fluid. Damming back the fluid further increases the intraventricular pressure.

Detailed *cerebral localization* is beyond the scope of this book, but gross area localization is important (130). The left hemisphere is the dominant one in a right handed individual; the right hemisphere, in a left handed person. The frontal lobes lie in front of the central sulci of Rolando. They are primarily motor. The parts immediately anterior to the central sulcus control voluntary muscular activity on the opposite side of the body (Fig. 285). The frontal and medial portions of the frontal lobe are concerned with such functions as psychic activity, cerebration, attention and judgment. Injury to or destruction of motor portions, results in contralateral hemiplegia whereas irritation will produce Jacksonian convulsions. Speech is initiated in the portion of the frontal lobe above the temporal lobe in the dominant hemisphere, and injury to this area will result in motor aphasia.

The parietal lobes which lie behind the frontal lobes and ahead of the occipital lobes are concerned with sensory reception for the contralateral half of the body. The anterior inferior parietal lobe in the dominant hemisphere controls visual or sensory speech. The occipital poles of the brain contain the visual centers (Fig. 285). Damage to this portion of the brain results in visual field loss to the opposite side. The temporal lobes in the dominant hemisphere are related to auditory speech, hearing, smell, and associated taste. A lesion deep in the temporal lobe will involve the optic radiations with loss of vision or visual hallucinations to the opposite side. The medial and basal structures of the brain, including the hypothalamus, thalamus, and mesencephalon, are concerned with vital functions such as blood pressure, respiration, metabolism, and temperature regulation.

CLINICAL SYMPTOMS

Craniocerebral injuries in children vary in severity with the stage of skull development and the force. Infants are frequently injured by falls from a bath table, high chair, bed, or the attendant's arms. There may be a period of unconsciousness lasting from a few seconds to minutes or hours. There may be a lucid interval followed by delayed stupor or unconsciousness, frequently indicating subdural or extradural hemorrhage. The duration of unconsciousness varies with the severity of the injury. Symptoms of pupillary change; motor paralysis; changing blood pressure, pulse and respiration are indicative of severe cerebral injury or hemorrhage. A rising temperature follows brain stem and hypothalamus injury. Rapidly increasing neurologic signs or symptoms should arouse suspicion of arterial hemorrhage. The depth and duration of unconsciousness are of prognostic value. Unconsciousness for days or weeks usually means serious cerebral damage and permanent symptoms, but injury to the tips of the frontal or temporal lobes may cause prolonged unconsciousness with ultimate complete recovery. Disorientation, restlessness and agitated tossing about are associated with laceration and hemorrhage of the inferior surfaces of the frontal and temporal lobes. Deep surgical shock, coma, and paralysis are indicative of cerebral laceration and hemorrhage. Extensor rigidity in which the head is thrown backward and the arms and legs rigidly extended with the hands flexed at the wrist and the feet plantar flexed may take place in severe cerebral laceration and hemorrhage with probable compression of the uncal portions of the temporal lobe on the brain stem at the tentorial opening.

The depth of unconsciousness is of immediate prognostic importance.

Failure to arouse from the stimulation of orbital pressure, deep muscle pressure or sphincter dilation is a grave sign. Response to such stimuli by defensive or purposeful movements, or the return of restless movements are more hopeful signs.

Increasing respiratory rate is an indication of severe cerebral damage with a poor prognosis. This is frequently associated with a rising temperature and increasing pulse rate. The rapid increase in pulse and respiratory rates is suggestive of intracerebral hemorrhage and mesencephalic failure. Sudden slowing of respirations or prolonged periods of apnea result from mesencephalic compression at the incisure of medullary compression at the foramen magnum rather than from hemorrhage within these structures.

An alarmingly *low pulse rate* and *rising blood pressure* are suggestive of an extradural or subdural blood clot. A slow pulse rate, forty to sixty per minute, may be physiologic for the patient but should be considered with other symptoms. It warrants close observation for changing or increasing neurologic signs. A rapid pulse following a slow pulse is a poor prognostic sign and indicates medullary failure. A sudden slowing of the pulse occurs in mass lesions, such as extradural or subdural hematomas with sudden compression effects.

Observation of the size and reaction of the pupils is very important for diagnosis and prognosis. Dilated, fixed or small contracted pupils are very unfavorable findings. A unilaterally dilated pupil occurs on the side of subdural or extradural hemorrhage, but may also occur as a result of injury to the optic nerve in a fracture of the orbit or sella turcica. A normal pupil which becomes dilated and fixed suggests extradural and subdural hemorrhage on the side of the dilated pupil, rarely on the opposite side. Papilledema, hemorrhages or choked discs seldom occur early in an injury unless there is a very large hematoma. Ocular paralysis usually occurs with gross hemorrhage or severe damage on the side of the paralysis. There may be bleeding or fluid drainage from the nose, mouth, or ears in basal skull fracture. Peripheral facial paralysis may occur in fractures of the petrous bone through the acoustic meatus and may be associated with hearing loss and bleeding or draining ear on the same side. Central facial paralysis in association with the paralysis of the arm or leg on the same side occurs in mass lesions on the opposite side of the brain.

It is often difficult to detect a *partial or complete paralysis* in a deeply unconscious patient. However, in a patient who can be aroused by external stimuli, failure of movement of one or more extremities may be significant of cerebral injury or hemorrhage. These changes are easily detected when the patient becomes restless and moves about. An extremity which does not move should be examined for evidence of fracture before it is moved by the examiner to detect paralysis. A paralyzed arm will fall flail when it is lifted and held above the face or chest whereas a non-paralyzed arm will fall more slowly with greater tone and a sliding effect. A leg that is paralyzed will flop to the side when it is flexed at the knee and hip and allowed to rest in that position. A non-paralyzed leg will rotate outward but at the same time it will slide to the extended position with definite muscle tone.

Convulsions following cerebral trauma may be significant of intracerebral or extracerebral hemorrhage, if there is no history of previous convulsions. Focal or Jacksonian convulsions which start in one extremity or muscle must make one think of a localized hematoma or an irritative lesion which requires operation.

MEDICAL TREATMENT

Common sense is the best prescription for medical management. Injury of the brain causes inhibited or depressed body function. Metabolic needs of the body should be met and natural body functions promoted. Adequate circulation is necessary for oxygenation of the brain. Unless he is in deep coma, an injured child finds a position which allows him the greatest comfort and freedom of body function. Nursing care must provide cleanliness and comfort for the patient even when he is semicomatose.

The treatment of shock by lowering the head, giving fluids, and stimulants, improves extracerebral circulation. The application of bandages or position of the head should not be allowed to obstruct the throat or compress the carotid arteries. A free air way must be maintained to allow adequate oxygen exchange in the lungs. Secretions in the throat, trachea or lungs, which interfere should be removed by aspiration, postural drainage or tracheotomy, as indicated. When oxygen is necessary, it is best administered in an oxygen tent. Many of the post traumatic cerebral residuals can be avoided by prompt correction of oxygen need. Restraints should be used only when absolutely necessary because even a semicomatose patient will fight them and in so doing raise his blood pressure, increase his oxygen need and counteract the benefit of other treatment.

The recognition and *treatment of other injuries* including skeletal and visceral are important in the treatment of craniocerebral injuries. Often the splinting of an injured extremity, emptying of a distended bladder, removal of a foreign body from a wound, or the application of a proper dressing will quiet a restless patient. The clothing may be irritating and harmfully stimulating and should be removed. The bed clothes and diapers should be clean, dry, and free of wrinkles.

Persistent restlessness is an indication of intracerebral or subarachnoidal bleeding. During the first twenty-four hours, mild barbiturate sedatives may be necessary to calm the patient. Pain in the craniocerebral injury is best relieved by aspirin. The use of narcotics cannot be too highly condemned in that they add depression to an already depressed brain. If pain is due to a fractured bone, injured muscle or viscus, and is not relieved by simple analgesics, stronger medication is necessary. Codeine in small doses is the safest drug. It should be limited to those cases in which it is urgently needed and in which cerebral depression is minimal.

Spinal puncture is not necessary as a diagnostic measure; the clinical signs are in themselves diagnostic. Lumbar puncture may temporarily relieve intracerebral pressure, but its effect is temporary and there is danger of promoting more bleeding. Spinal puncture in the first twelve or twenty-four hours in the presence of a large intra or extracerebral hematoma may produce a pressure cone at the incisura.

Lumbar punctures may be a valuable adjunct in the management of craniocerebral injuries and skull fractures, but must be used cautiously. Blood in the spinal fluid acts as a meningeal irritant with resulting restlessness and mild neck rigidity. Removal of bloody fluid is sometimes necessary, but should be postponed for twenty-four hours, if expedient.

The intravenous injection of *strongly hypertonic solutions* is no longer routine. While such solutions have been shown to reduce intracranial pressure and brain volume, the after effect is to increase both of these above the original level. Hypertonic solutions do not decompress the brain in the presence of punctuate hemorrhages.

Food and fluid intake should meet physiologic requirements. Dehydration and starvation are not only contraindicated, but are definitely harmful. Fluids can be administered by mouth, intravenously or subcutaneously, to maintain normal urine concentration and moisture of the mucous membranes. If the patient cannot take food by mouth, it can be given to him in liquid form through a small nasal catheter.

ACTIVITY

It is now generally conceded that the patient should be allowed to change position following an injury. He may roll from side to side and sit upright. Change of posture helps to maintain vasomotor stability and prevents many of the sequelae of vasomotor instability. Walking or jarring should be avoided for at least two weeks in the more serious cases. Such precaution is then unnecessary, as tissue healing is adequate to withstand ordinary activities.

SURGICAL TREATMENT

Many cases of craniocerebral injury require some surgical treatment varying from local scalp repair to major craniotomy (Fig. 286). Each case

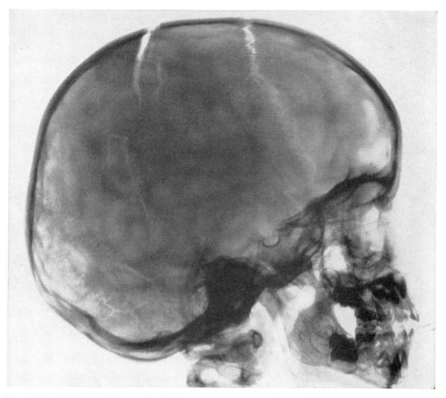

FIG. 286. Multiple linear skull fractures are not of necessity serious, but the patient must be watched for cerebral symptoms.

is individual and dogmatic rules cannot be given to guide treatment. One of the most neglected surgical needs in craniocerebral injuries in both children and adults is the maintenance of an *adequate air way*. If the exchange of air to the lungs is hindered by obstruction that cannot be relieved otherwise, a tracheotomy should be performed early and maintained until the need is completely past. *Adequate oxygenation* of an injured brain is essential and may be the factor which will prevent dire post traumatic sequelae.

Scalp wounds constitute by far the largest number of injuries requiring surgical treatment. No scalp wound, regardless of how trivial its appearance, should be neglected. The hair is clipped and the scalp shaved widely. The wound is thoroughly cleansed with surgical soap and repaired under local anesthesia, if possible. Hemostasis is best obtained by digital pressure with the tips of the fingers on each side of the wound. The wound edges are spread with the fingers and the area inspected and palpated for fracture or contamination. The contused devitalized scalp is thoroughly debrided and closed in layers (Fig. 287). If there is a fracture without depression or displacement the wound is closed as above described.

Major operations should be carried out with specialized neurosurgical

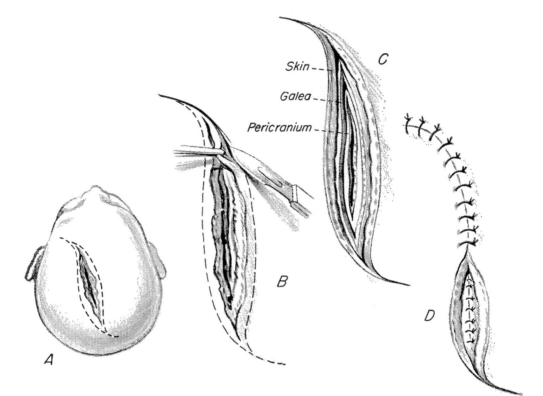

Fig. 287. Scalp laceration and repair. A. Outline of the "S" flap. B. Careful debridement of the contused skin edges. C. The skull is inspected for a fracture. A dirty wound has been converted to a clean one. D. Tight closure in layers without drainage in the fresh case. [Modified from Bancroft and Pilcher (129).]

equipment and technic. No major surgical procedures could be carried out without an electro-surgical unit, suction apparatus, Cushing clips, bone wax, cranial burs, rongeurs, retractors, and methods for hemostasis.

The *principles of treatment of open depressed fractures of the skull* (Fig. 289) are those of open fractures elsewhere in the body (Chapter XVI). A painstaking debridement and repair should be carried out only by one skilled in such surgery. Prior to the days of chemotherapy and antibiotics, the surgical repair of a compound depressed skull fracture was an emergency procedure that had to be finished within the first twelve hours. Prompt repair is still advisable, but surgical wisdom now demands that the patient be brought to the best possible condition before surgical repair is carried out, even though twenty-four hours may elapse.

The fresh scalp wound is made into a clean wound by removal of contaminated and contused tissue (Fig 287). Depressed bone fragments that can be lifted out without difficulty are removed (Fig. 288). If there is the slightest question of contamination they are discarded. One should never

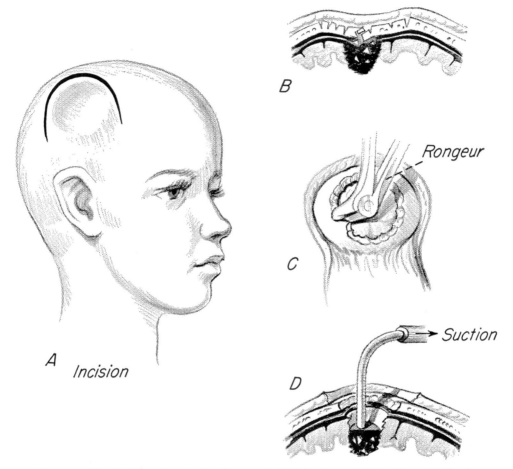

FIG. 288. Surgical treatment of a depressed skull fracture. A. Skin flap with the base caudad to expose the fracture. B. Diagramatic representation of the depression, the bone fragments and brain damage. C. Removal of the depressed fragments. D. Removal of necrotic tissue, foreign bodies, and blood by suction.

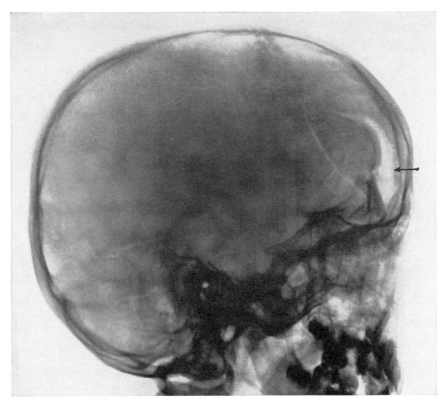

Fig. 289. M. B., male, age 7, 9/15/53. Lateral view of an open comminuted depressed frontal skull fracture.

elevate the depressed fragments blindly. When these fragments cannot be easily removed, a bur hole is placed at the edge of the depression, the depressed area thoroughly encircled with a rongeur, and the fragments lifted out carefully. In this way, tears in the dura and brain can readily be seen and properly handled. When the dura has been penetrated, the bone fragments are gently extracted and the dural rent is opened more widely to allow thorough inspection of the brain. Bleeding vessels are coagulated and the contused brain is debrided by suction and irrigation. The dura is closed water tight and the scalp wound sutured in anatomic layers. Clean bone may be replaced in the cranial defect (Fig. 290).

Closed depressed fractures should be elevated. The depression is always greater than appears in roentgenograms. The timing depends upon the patient's condition. Depressed fractures seldom require immediate surgical correction. They can be treated as elective procedures and wait for skilled neurosurgical management.

Derby hat or rubber ball skull depression sometimes occurs in a newborn from forceps pressure or intrauterine impingement against a bony

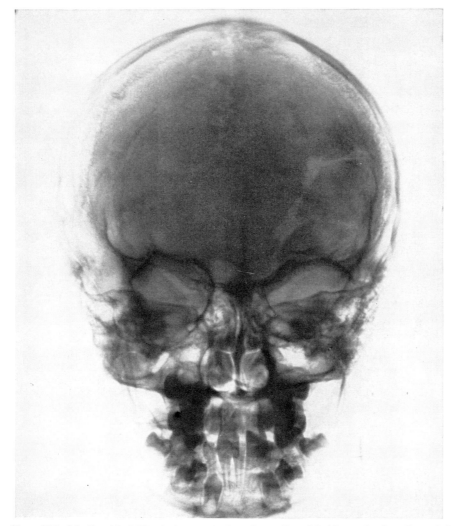

FIG. 290. M. B., 10/6/53. Anteroposterior view after debridement, elevation of the fragments to the normal contour.

prominence. The indentation rarely causes neurologic disturbance and usually reduces itself spontaneously within ten days. Gentle pressure around the borders of the depressed area will often mold the depression back to normal contour. If the depression persists longer than ten days, surgical correction may be necessary. The safest method is to work through a bur opening at the edge of the depression. A curved elevator is inserted between the depressed bone and the dura and the depressed area gently elevated (Fig. 291).

Hemorrhage resulting from trauma to the head may be extradural, subdural, subarachnoid or intracerebral. *Extradural bleeding* usually occurs

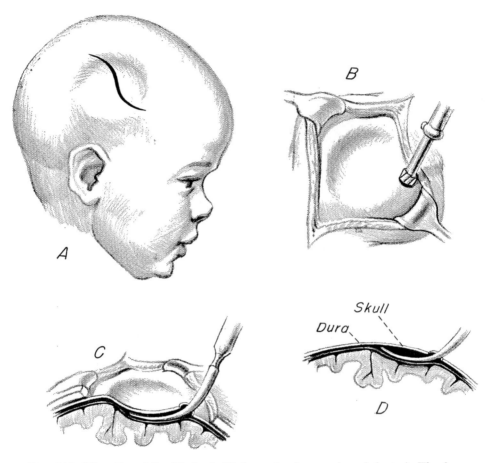

FIG. 291. Elevation of the "derby hat" depression in a newborn infant. A. The depression with the overlying skin incision. B. Trephine hole at the edge of the depression. C. Insertion of the curved elevator between the skull and the dura. D. Elevation of the skull into normal position.

in the middle fossa of the skull following a tear of the middle meningeal artery by a fracture of the temporal bone. This arterial hemorrhage is viscious in its persistence. Unless it is recognized early and operated upon promptly it results in rapid loss of consciousness, contralateral paralysis, and death. One must remove an adequate amount of bone to allow aspiration of the hematoma and coagulation, clipping or ligation of the offending vessel.

Subdural bleeding is usually the result of a tear of a vein running from the cortex to a venous sinus. Although the bleeding may be profuse, the pressure of the brain and hematoma against the bleeding vessel may stop the bleeding temporarily or permanently (Fig. 292). A large subdural hematoma produces symptoms promptly. Days, weeks or months may

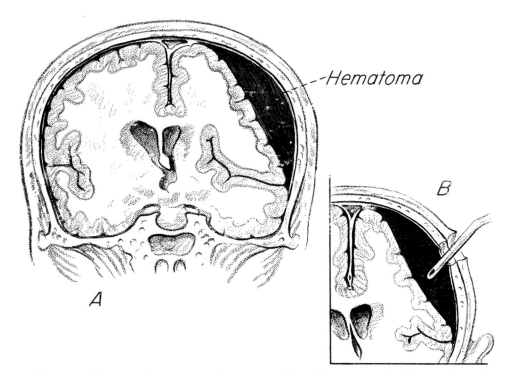

FIG. 292. Diagramatic representation of a subdural hematoma. A. Compression of the hemisphere with displacement of the ventricles to the opposite side. B. Craniotomy for removal of the hematoma. [Redrawn from Bancroft and Pilcher (129).]

pass before further bleeding takes place or before the encapsulated hematoma draws in fluid by osmotic pressure to enlarge it into a compressing, paralyzing or irritating lesion. Subdural hygroma is a collection of cerebrospinal fluid that escaped through a tear of the arachnoid into the subdural space. The fluid becomes xanthochromic with an increase in protein because of the stasis or associated bleeding. The symptoms of chronic subdural hygroma or hemorrhage are restlessness, irritability, vomiting, weight loss, convulsions, and occasional weakness or paralysis. Headaches are almost invariable and are due to blood vessel or sinus traction by the blood clot or hygroma.

The diagnosis of subdural hematoma or hygroma may be made by subdural puncture in the infant with patent fontanels. The collection of blood or fluid should be removed surgically, however, rather than by repeated aspiration. If the fontanels are closed and subdural hemorrhage is suspected cerebral arteriograms, pneumoencephalogram or trephine exploration may be necessary for diagnosis. When the diagnosis has been established, an osteoplastic craniotomy is necessary as in an adult for removal of the fluid (Fig. 292B).

Subarachnoid hemorrhage due to injury to a cortical vessel may remain in the subarachnoid space or extend into one of the spinal fluid cisterns. Irritation from the blood or its components may simulate meningitis.

Intracerebral hemorrhage is usually diffuse, and rarely localized enough to permit surgical removal. Hemorrhage into the brain stem produces grave disturbances of vital functions.

Subtemporal decompression operations are not to be used indiscriminately for the relief of post traumatic increased intracranial pressure and edema. Even in the hands of the most skillful neurologic surgeon, this procedure adds trauma to an already injured brain. Herniation of the brain takes place at the site of the decompression and produces a ringlike swelling and edema at the point of herniation with additional brain damage.

Cranioplasty. Defects in the skull following loss of bone in open or open depressed skull fractures seldom need covering in infants or children. Since sutures or fixed attachments to the skull may prevent its normal growth, the material used to cover a skull defect in a child must not be attached to the skull. When a defect is potentially dangerous enough to requre protection, a large plastic or tantalum plate to overlay the defect on all sides, can be fixed satisfactorily to the soft tissue to prevent is displacement.

CHAPTER XVI

Open (Compound) Fractures

GENERAL PRINCIPLES

Modern transportation produces open fractures in children which are similar to those of adults. The treatment is the same with regard to thorough cleansing and immediate debridement of the wound. One who treats the fracture must evaluate the soft tissue injury and be prepared to deal with tendon and nerve laceration. For discussion of the subject see Chapter VI, Injuries of the Hand.

Internal fixation is frequently necessary in the immobilization of adult bones that must be accurately reduced and securely held. The rules for children are different. There is rarely need for internal fixation. Usually one can debride the wound and apply a simple cast. Skeletal traction with a Kirschner wire incorporated in a cast distal to the wound may be used if there is considerable comminution or loss of bone substance (Fig. 293). In children the ability to bridge bone defects is indirectly proportional to the age, and nonunion is rare. Some shortening is not only permissible but desirable. The stimulus of the healing fracture with the addition of the inflammatory reaction about the healing soft part wound, will cause considerable overgrowth (Fig. 294). Accelerated growth is likely to continue longer if there is local infection.

Internal fixation is justifiable in children only when it would be mechanically necessary were it a closed fracture like one of the lateral humeral condyle. When used, pins should be removed. A plate with screws is generally bad. It is likely to break. If left in a child it is either inert and is completely buried in the bone so that it is very difficult to remove later, or there is considerable reaction with prolonged overgrowth. The bone under a plate may be weakened enough to give rise to a pathologic fracture.

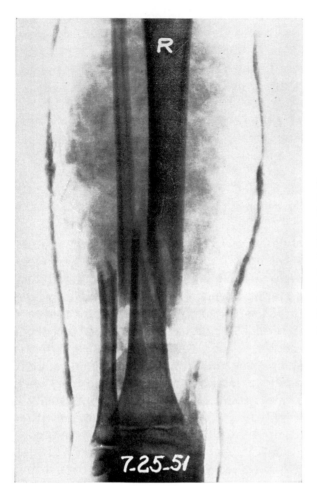

FIG. 293. G. G., male, age 7. An open fracture of both bones of the right leg was associated with extensive soft tissue damage. Immediate careful debridement and partial closure. A Kirschner wire through the heel was incorporated in a plaster cast. The roentgenogram was taken six days after the injury. The foot was elevated in bed on traction. Note the bayonet apposition and the shortening of about 15 mm.

An open fracture is a true surgical emergency. Minutes are precious. The fractured bone should be splinted at the site of the accident and the child taken at once to a hospital where definitive treatment can be carried out. Protruding bone ends should not be pulled back into the wound. Innocent looking puncture wounds have been responsible for death from gas gangrene. The compound fracture incident to the child's play is usually contaminated with dirt which harbors the spores of tetanus and gas gangrene. The contamination of the wounds of highway accidents needs no comment.

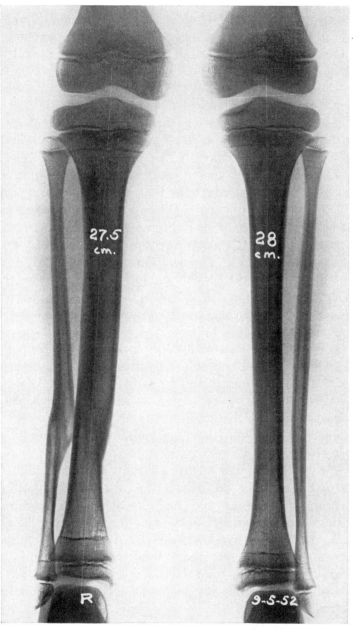

FIG. 294. G. G. Anteroposterior view of both legs one year after the preceding roentgenogram. Molding had almost eliminated the local deformity which was not evident clinically. Accelerated growth had made up all but 5 mm. of the shortening on the right. Note the lines of growth at the ends of the tibiae which clearly demonstrate the acceleration of growth. The gain all occurred in the first five months. No further equalization was anticipated.

EMERGENCY TREATMENT

A roentgenogram should be taken through the splint and the child transferred immediately to the operating room. Preparation is carried out with the technical precaution observed in a major operation. A protruding bone end is covered with a sponge and the surrounding area is cleansed with a detergent or a bland soap and copious amounts of sterile water or saline. If hair is present the part is shaved. With sterile glove technic the wound itself is then cleansed. If the bone end is dirty, it is removed with a rongeur. No antiseptic is used. Most of the unfortunate complications of compound fractures are due to delay and dirt. The surgeon trims away contused wound margins and devitalized soft tissue. Compound wounds of children require the excision of less tissue than those of adults because the recuperative power is greater, but the prompt debridement of a crushed wound is important.

After changing gloves, the surgeon reduces the fracture by traction and a minimum of manipulation. The wound may be enlarged for inspection of the bone ends. It should be thoroughly cleansed with detergents and many rinsings of saline after the reduction. Exact timing of the procedure is ridiculous but the wound toilet will consume not less than one-half hour in a complicated case.

If there is only the tip of a small splinter of bone protruding through a minute clean wound which was obviously produced from the inside out by the spicule itself, it is sufficient to thoroughly cleanse and/or remove the protruding tip and pull it back into position. There is very little likelihood of contamination of such a wound, but in all cases, *antibiotics* should be started immediately. After these preliminaries, the fracture may be treated as a closed one.

A booster shot of *toxoid, or tetanus antiotxin* (not gas bacillus) must be given. The dosage depends on the local conditions and not the age of the child. In administering antitoxins, one cannot do better than follow the advice of the Committee for the Study of Immunization as Prophylaxis for Tetanus and Gas Gangrene (131). "As regards immunization with tetanus antitoxin: For wounds seen within twenty-four hours after injury the usual dose of antitoxin shall be 1,500 units. For a large wound or known gross contamination, the prophylactic dose of antitoxin shall be 3,000 units.

"For wounds, seen later than twenty-four hours after injury the indicated dosage of antitoxin should be doubled for each day of elapsed time up to a total of 10,000 units.

"For wounds not susceptible to adequate surgical debridement, containing residual devitalized tissue or remaining unhealed there is an obligation to prolong the period of protection with antitoxin. The preferred procedure is to repeat the administration of 1,500 units of antitoxin every seven days until the wound is clean or healed. An alternatively acceptable method is to administer a larger dose (up to 100,000 units) initially with the expectation that the larger dose will provide a longer period (up to three weeks) of passive protection. The use of tetanus antiotoxin should always be preceded by appropriate and meticulously performed tests for sensitivity to horse protein. The tetanus antitoxin must be diluted 1:10 in saline solution for intracutaneous or ophthalmic testing. Only a minute amount of the diluted material should be put into the eye or the skin. The skin wheal should be about the size of the head of a pin lest false positives occur when larger quantities are injected. When both eye and skin tests are positive, the danger of anaphylaxis is greater than the hazard of tetanus. The facts about serum reactions may be summarized as follows: (1) Negative tests render immediate serum reactions unlikely, but fatal anaphylactic reactions have occurred after negative skin and eye tests. (2) Negative tests have no pertenency as regards vulnerability to delayed serum reactions occurring up to ten days after administration of antitoxin. (3) The incidence and severity of reactions are greatest with intrathecal and intravenous serum, and least with intramuscular serum. (4) Positive skin tests, a previous dose of antitoxin or known sensitivity to horse proteins render serum therapy dangerous. It has not been proven that desensitization programs for administration of serum are capable of providing antitoxin immunity. (5) In the event equine antitoxin is contraindicated, bovine antitoxin should be used after appropriate skin tests are shown to be negative. (6) Adequate prophylaxis for serum reactions may be defined as: (a) administration of 0.3 ml. of 1:1000 adrenaline in an oily base immediately prior to the injection of antitoxin; (b) antihistamine drugs for ten days. (7) Adequate treatment for an established serum reaction is provided with ACTH."

If toxoid is used the "basic, or initial, vaccination should be achieved by the use of slowly absorbed alum precipitated toxoid. Combination of alum tetanus toxoid with either diphtheria toxoid, pertussis vaccine or typhoid vaccine is not only satisfactory but appears to be desirable.

"Routine booster doses are best given as alum precipitated toxoid. Wound booster doses of toxoid are best given as the more rapidly absorbed fluid toxoid.

"After the lapse of more than four years after the last booster dose of toxoid there is often a delayed or inadequate response to toxoid beyond the four to five day period usually required for the recall of antitoxic antibodies."

Tetanus antitoxin and toxoid should be used at the same time in "individuals not previously vaccinated with toxoid and receiving tetanus

antitoxin, active immunization with toxoid should be started concomitantly because the sensitizing effect of the prophylactic serum renders subsequent antitoxin therapy hazardous and uncertain. Toxoid should be 1
ml. in quantity, given in a separate syringe and at a separate site.

"In individuals previously vaccinated with toxoid, although the mat-
ter is controversial, the coincident use of toxoid and antitoxin may be
considered whenever: (1) A massively contaminated wound and delayed
surgical care create the hazard of likely onset of tetanus prior to the lapse
of a further four to five days required for response to toxoid. (2) The lapse
of more than four years from the time of the last booster dose produces a
situation wherein a small but definite group of previously vaccinated patients require six or more days for response to toxoid."

In the prophylaxis of gas gangrene, antitoxin is ineffective and is not
recommended. "Gas gangrene toxoids show experimental promise but
await clinical evaluation. The most reliable prophylaxis of gas gangrene
is early and adequate wound surgery (debridement) with the wound
being left open. Several days later, when the wound is clean, it may be
closed by delayed suture."

The question of *closure of contaminated wounds* is one that requires
considerable judgment. It is wiser to leave fifty wounds open than to close
one with the inclusion of foreign material which causes a serious infection.
There are so many factors operating that dogmatic rules cannot be laid
down. If the compound wound is fresh, relatively clean, and incised rather
than crushed, it may well be closed. When there is a delay of several hours,
a large wound with crushing of the soft parts should be packed open with
vaseline. At most, the ends may be closed for a short distance. Between
these extremes various courses may be followed. The loose closure of
many fresh, open, but clean fractures is permissible in children.

Open fractures of the femur with minimal soft tissue damage may be
placed in traction like closed fractures. If there is extensive damage, it is
better to use a cast combined with skeletal traction applied to the crest
of the tibia for more complete immobilization. When soft part healing is
delayed, it is a good plan to continue the plaster cast even after the bones
have united. In children there is little danger of joint stiffness from prolonged immobilization. Constant movement near a joint will perpetuate
a residual spot of granulation for weeks.

PROGNOSIS

The prognosis for open fractures in children differs from that in adults
in several ways. The growth factor contributes greatly to the end result
(Fig. 294). A bone which is short may be stimulated to accelerated growth
and be longer than its fellow at the termination of the growth period. The

degree of bone disruption is a rough index of the amount of overgrowth that will occur. The nearness to the epiphyseal plate is of little, if any, significance. If the fracture or a subsequent infection involves the epiphyseal plate there may be shortening and/or angular deformity.

LATE TREATMENT

Sequestrum formation is less frequent in children than in adults because of the more rapid revascularization of devitalized bone. It is wise to wait for several months before deciding to remove a piece of dead bone (Fig. 296, p. 256). Frequently the wound will heal and the dead bone absorb. When there is persistent drainage about a sequestrum, the latter should be removed if the surrounding new bone is strong enough to support the extremity. The closed plaster technic with the application of a vaseline drain is desirable in such cases. Primary closure is sometimes feasible if one can be sure of antibiotic coverage.

When there is a large area of *granulation tissue*, prompt healing may be obtained by the use of split thickness graft taken from the same extremity or from the opposite thigh. Healing is more rapid than in adults, however, and surprisingly large defects will heal spontaneously.

Pathologic Fractures

ETIOLOGY

Pathologic fractures are those which occur with minimal trauma because a bone is weakened by some abnormal condition. The deficiency of the bone may be due to local changes or may be a part of a generalized skeletal disease. "Spontaneous fractures" of apparently normal bones in children are limited to fatigue fractures (march fractures) (Fig. 295). They are not actually "spontaneous", but are caused by some unusual activity, repeated so many times that the bone fatigues and breaks.

True pathologic fractures occur in children from different causes than in adults. Paget's disease, senile atrophy, and Charcot's disease, which weaken so many bones in adults, are not found in children. Metastatic malignancy is an unusual cause of fracture. Excessive radiation therapy causes epiphyseal damage with subsequent deformity in the growing child but rarely causes bone necrosis and fracture. In children, on the other hand we encounter congenital fractures, osteogenesis imperfecta, and slipped femoral epiphyses (Chapter VII, Injuries of the Femur) which do not occur in adults.

FRACTURES DUE TO LOCAL CAUSES

Local atrophy of bone may be due to prolonged postoperative immobilization. It is rare in children except in combination with an inflammatory process such as tuberculosis or osteomyelitis (Fig. 296); or a neurologic deficit as found in chronic poliomyelitis or spina bifida. In such cases, the prolonged immobilization of a bone which is already atrophic leads to extreme and sometimes disastrous bone atrophy with frequent fractures without actual trauma (Fig. 297). Premature closure of the epiphyses (132) is part of the same process. Pathologic fractures associated with the atrophic bones of poliomyelitis heal readily. Since there is very little soft tissue injury, pain is slight and the fracture may go unrecognized. Fractures associated with sensory as well as motor paralysis (spina bifida) may be entirely painless. They are well treated with traction. Exuberant callus appears in unbelievable amounts (Fig. 298).

Benign cystic bone lesions contribute the greatest number of pathologic fractures in children (Fig. 299A). Bone cysts of the proximal ends of the humerus, femur, and tibia, less frequently elsewhere in long bones, are usually unrecognized until the fracture occurs. There is very little pain when the extremity is at rest. The etiology is obscure. Simple bone cysts are usually classified as neoplasms, but they may be only evidence of injury and repair. The diagnosis can usually be made from the roentgenogram. It is confirmed by microscopic study of the membrane lining the cavity.

The treatment of the fracture consists of immobilization with traction or a cast. Fracture of the proximal end of the humerus is well managed with a hanging cast. Healing is prompt. This fact has led to some confusion in the literature. While the fracture heals, the cysts rarely disappear completely and permanently except in the adolescent. As a rule the cyst reforms and a succession of fractures results.

After the fracture heals, the accepted orthopaedic treatment is eradication of the cyst and packing of the cavity with bone chips. Recurrence after this treatment is not infrequent even if excision is carried well beyond the ends of the cyst (Fig. 299B). It makes little difference whether autogenous bone or homogenous bone from the bank be used for packing. It is doubtful whether the results are better following cautery of the cavity with phenol flushed out by alcohol.

Beginning recurrence of the cyst may be effectively treated by radiation. This is safe if the lesion is near the center of a long bone. Frequently the lesion is near the epiphyseal plate and radiation carries a considerable hazard of growth retardation. Roentgen therapy should not be given before the diagnosis is established by biopsy.

The study of cases of bone cyst during the entire growth period has shown that the cysts disappear spontaneously at puberty. This is true whether the cyst has been operated upon or not. Proof of this fact may be obtained indirectly from a review of cases in any large orthopaedic clinic. One rarely, if ever, obtains a history of multiple fractures through the proximal end of the humerus due to bone cyst in a child, with persistence of the fracture in the adult patient. Pathologic fractures due to similar bone cysts in adults start during adult life and are not carry overs from children's bone cysts.

With the fact in mind that bone cysts heal spontaneously at puberty, it is logical to treat these pathologic fractures conservatively in older children who may never have a second fracture. This is particularly true of girls. Even though they have a second fracture, the result may be more pleasing than a scar. Young boys would be greatly incapacitated by multiple fractures and should have an operation to eradicate the cyst and pack with bone chips. The curettement should be carried well beyond the end of the cyst in both directions. Care must be exercised to avoid injuring an epiphyseal plate. Cauterization is not necessary. Packing with bone chips hastens restoration of the strength of the bone. Homogenous bone is useful for this purpose.

Fibrous dysplasia of bone is sometimes similar in appearance and is not differentiated from simple cyst in most text books. *Monostotic fibrous dysplasia* usually appears in the roentgenogram as a fusiform enlargement of the bone with irregularity of density (Fig. 300). There may be several small translucent areas or there may be one large one. In the latter case, the differential diagnosis from bone cyst is sometimes difficult. Usually the outlines of the translucent area are irregular and ill defined. There is a lacy appearance of the margins. The bone surrounding the cystic lesion is usually more abnormal than in bone cyst.

Fracture through the fibrous lesion is frequently unknown to the patient. An unexplained limp or weakness of an arm may bring him in for examination. An incomplete fracture in the roentgenogram will then call attention to a lesion. If untreated the fracture frequently heals in deformity and refracture occurs when activity is resumed.

The differential diagnosis must be made following a biopsy and microscopic examination. Complete eradication of the cystic areas and packing with bone chips usually leads to prompt healing. Deformity can be corrected at a later operation after the diagnosis is established, frequently in combination with the excision of a recurrent focus (Fig. 301).

The preceding two entities should not be confused with small *non-ossifying cortical fibromas* (141) which disappear spontaneously with growth and do not give rise to pathologic fracture (Fig. 225, p. 178).

Hemangioma of bone causes a cystic lesion which may fracture (Fig. 302). The cyst is usually multilocular. The operative treatment is much more difficult than that of simple bone cyst. While the lesion is benign there is a strong tendency to recurrence. The extreme vascularity makes operative removal exceedingly difficult. Replacement of blood is necessary. If a tourniquet is not feasible, temporary occlusion of the main arterial supply is imperative.

Hemangioma of bone usually reveals itself as a bony enlargement before the fracture takes place. The roentgenogram shows the appearance of many bubbles which is characteristic. The first fracture will heal satisfactorily but the lesion usually progresses locally. Complete resection and replacement with a bone graft is usually necessary and should be done before the lesion becomes too large. There is no objection to performing this resection at the time of the fracture. In this it differs from bone cysts in which it is expedient to operate for eradication of the cyst when the fracture is healed.

Multiple hemangiomas of bone offer a problem which is still insoluble (Fig. 303). They may occur in many bones simultaneously (Fig. 304). One cannot resect all of the bones. The fractures must be treated as they occur, much like those of osteogenesis imperfecta.

Aneurysmal bone cysts, a rare cause of fracture, occur in children and young adults, usually under twenty. Originally called 'giant cell tumors' they are eccentric swellings of the bone with a thin shell, coarse trabeculations of the base of the cyst and fine trabeculations in the lesion itself. The spaces are full of blood rather than clear fluid. Curettage usually effects a complete cure. The prognosis is good and radiation therapy is usually not indicated (133, 134).

Congenital fracture of the tibia (localized neurofibromatosis). A child may be born with a pseudarthrosis of the tibia as a result of localized neurofibromatosis. A similar fracture may occur during infancy usually at the site of an angular deformity of the bone with the apex anteriorly (Fig. 305). The circumference of the bone is usually diminished at the site of the angulation with obliteration of the medulla so that the bone is characteristically small and sclerotic. Small translucent areas may or may not be present.

If the bone is not already broken through, but angulated with the apex anteriorly, an ill-advised osteotomy or osteoclasis characteristically terminates in a nonunion. The prognosis in a spontaneous fracture is the same. Massive bone grafts when they remain successful until after puberty give a better result than amputation. Refracture with persistent pseudarthrosis is common in childhood (135). Amputation is to be preferred to permanent pseudarthrosis. New hope is offered with the use of Sofield's method of serial section of the affected bone with intramedullar fixation (Fig. 306) (138).

Fatigue fractures (march fractures) have been discussed, as they occur in the metatarsals in children (Chapter X, Injuries of the Foot). As in adults, almost any long bone might be involved, but the tibia is next in frequency (Fig. 295). Fatigue fracture of this bone appears following sustained exertion in older boys.

The cause is not entirely clear. The fracture may be due to repeated bending of the bone which finally fatigues and breaks much as a metal rod will break with similar treatment. It may be that fatigue leads to vascular spasm and local necrosis of bone which predisposes to fracture under excessive strain.

The diagnosis should be suspected when there is a sudden onset of tenderness and swelling over both the dorsal and volar surfaces of the distal end of the second or third metatarsal. Pain, swelling, and tenderness may be present for a week before there is any roentgenologic evidence of either fracture or callus. The callus may appear before the fracture line. If a roentgenogram is taken in ten days, the fracture will usually be evident. Later, massive callus is somewhat suggestive of a sarcoma. Legs have been sacrificed by amputation because a fatigue fracture was wrongly diagnosed as a malignant tumor.

FRACTURES DUE TO GENERALIZED ABNORMALITIES

Generalized atrophy of the bones of a child may be idiopathic (136). Severe rickets which is now rarely seen in enlightened communities will cause a similar predisposition to fracture. It is analagous to osteomalacia in adults.

Osteogenesis imperfecta is a generalized hypoplasia of the skeleton associated with multiple spontaneous fractures (Fig. 307). The fragility of of the bones is due to a defect in development rather than the inability of the patient to assimilate calcium and phosphorus, as shown by the normal metabolism of these elements. Key (137) recognizes three types: (1) Osteogenesis imperfecta associated with fractures at or soon after birth without actual trauma. (2) Idiopathic osteopsathyrosis in which the fractures do not occur until after the patient begins to walk. These cases have blue sclerae and the bones are slender and brittle. (3) Hereditary hypoplasia of the mesenchyme is like the second except that it is transmitted as a dominant hereditary factor and the affected individuals have a tendency to develop deafness in early adult life.

True osteogenesis imperfecta is frequently fatal during the first few years of life. If the child survives there is a tendency to improvement and the bony abnormality may clear up at puberty leaving in its wake, multiple deformities. Moderate bowing of the femurs and tibias can be corrected by osteoclasis with immobilization by traction or a cast. The difficulty is that the contracted soft parts prevent correction of extreme deformities by this means. Open operation is then necessary. Children with this disease stand shock very poorly and fatalities have been reported.

The chief drawback to the correction of deformity is that the child will refracture the same bone again promptly on being allowed even restricted activity. A most ingenious and effective method of overcoming this difficulty has recently been developed by Dr. Harold Sofield (Figs. 308, 309).

Complete subperiosteal exposure of the bone and resection from metaphysis to metaphysis permits the segmental section of the bone like thick slices of sausage. These slices are all strung on an intramedullary nail; the central ones rotated so as to reverse the deformity. They are replaced with the intramedullary nail engaged in either metaphysis. Healing is prompt with elimination of deformity (Fig. 309). The intramedullary nail is left in situ to prevent displacement if further fracture occurs. The incidence of fracture is greatly diminished by the internal support. In some cases the rod has been replaced when the bone grows too long for it (138).

Eosinophilic granuloma and other disorders of the reticuloendothelial system must be differentiated from osteomyelitis or bone tumors. Pathologic fracture may be the first indication that the lesion is present (Fig. 310). Usually there is pain, swelling, and systemic involvement including a low fever and rapid sedimentation rate. Involvement of a single vertebra may be the cause of some cases of Calvé's disease (Chapter XIII, Injuries of the Spine).

Infantile scurvy is characterized by several types of pathologic fractures. The brittle metaphyses may split or be compressed to a cup shape (139). In the severe cases, epiphyseal displacement at the ends of long bones occurs (Fig. 311). All types of pathologic fractures heal rapidly under appropriate medical treatment with adequate orange juice. The shaft of the bone aligns itself with the new position of the epiphysis and deformity is almost unknown. The patient's posture in bed usually corrects the alignment. Gross angular distortions should be corrected.

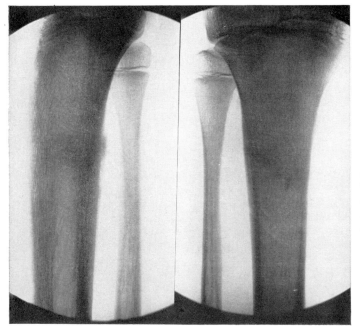

FIG. 295. March Fracture

R. C., male, age 14. March fracture of the proximal end of the tibia appearing in the early days of basketball season. Swelling and tenderness over the site of the fracture. The roentgenogram was taken about ten days after the onset of symptoms. Complete recovery with rest. (Courtesy of Dr. John Pink.)

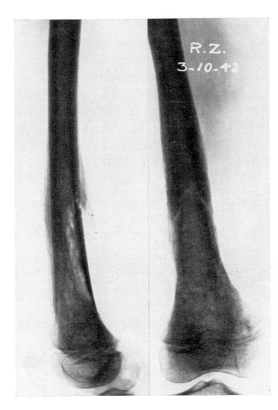

Fig. 296. Chronic Osteomyelitis

R. Z., male. Pathologic fracture of the distal end of the femur through the site of a hematogenous osteomyelitis. Immobilization in a plaster cast with healing. The sequestrum which was visible in the lateral view separated entirely and then absorbed without open operation. Complete healing with antibiotic treatment but the bone grew too long. (Courtesy of Dr. A. C. Schmidt.)

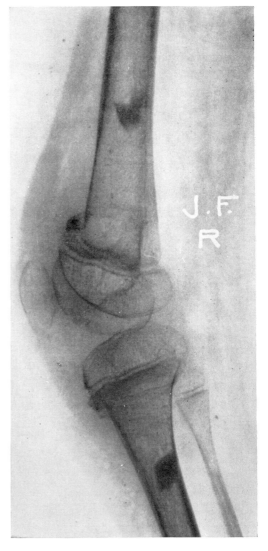

Fig. 297. Spontaneous Fracture

J. F., female, age 12, 7/27/53. Extreme bone atrophy due to neurotrophic disturbance associated with spina bifida, plus postoperative immobilization following a hip operation. "Spontaneous" fractures through the metaphyses of the femur and tibia occurred while the patient walked on crutches. The dense shadows were ivory, used for stimulation of growth.

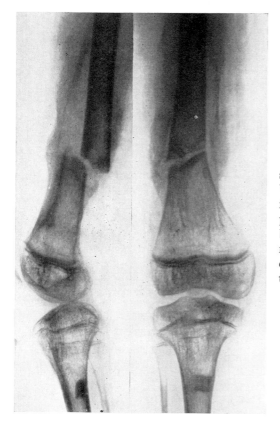

FIG. 298. Neurotrophic Callus

J. F., 4/6/54. The case illustrated in Figure 297 shows healing of the previous metaphyseal fractures. With minimal trauma the patient fractured the femur completely at a higher level. There was no pain. While on traction the patient moved freely in bed producing the tremendous callus seen in the roentgenogram. Healing was very prompt as it frequently is in bones which are subject to a neurotrophic atrophy.

FIG. 299. Bone Cyst

A. W.C., 4/23/47, male, age 10. Pathologic fracture of the right humerus through a bone cyst. With a hanging cast, the fracture healed but the cyst did not disappear. The cyst was completely eradicated and packed with bone chips from the ilium on 8/25/47. The diagnosis was confirmed microscopically. The cyst reformed and was curetted again on 4/2/48 and packed with chips from the bank. B. 11/10/48. Note the growth of the humerus proximal to the cyst. Roentgen therapy to the area but cystic areas remained until the child reached maturity, when they disappeared. This sequence of events is typical.

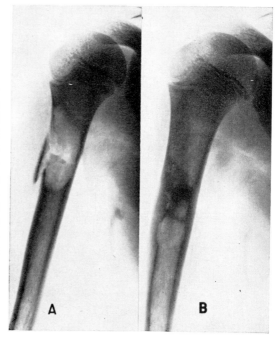

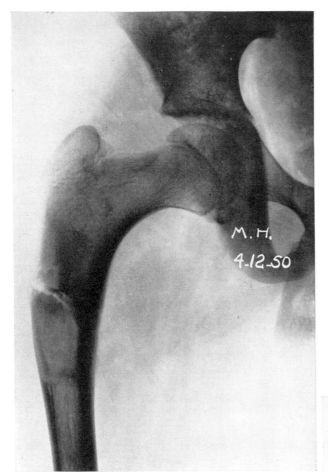

Fig. 300. Monostatic Fibrous
Dysplasia

M. H., male, age 14. Incomplete
fracture of the proximal end of the
right femur through a monostotic
fibrous dysplasia. Five years previously there had been a similar
fracture which healed completely but
with the neck of the femur in varus.
Intermittent limp since, aggravated
recently without the patient knowing
about the present fracture. A biopsy
was performed, the cystic lesion
curetted, and packed with bone chips.

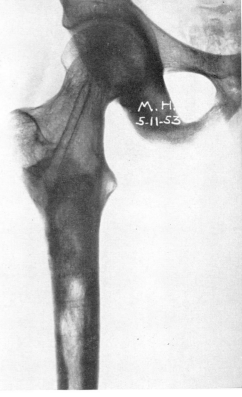

Fig. 301. M. H., 5/11/53. After the lesion shown
in Figure 300 had healed, an osteotomy was performed to correct the coxa vara. At the same time a
small recurrent cystic area was curetted. Internal
fixation with a blade plate. The hardware was removed on 2/12/53. This roentgenogram was taken
three months after the last operation. No limp. No
complaint. Hip motions symmetrical. There was 1
cm. of shortening of the right leg.

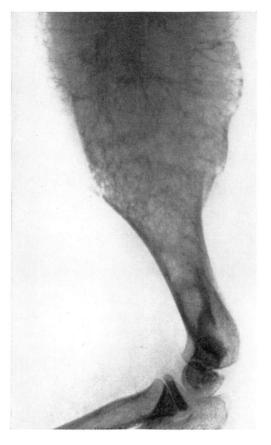

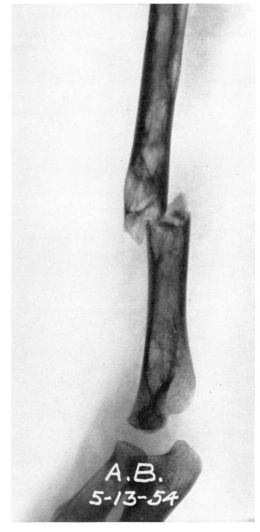

FIG. 302. Solitary Hemangioma

Male, age 8. Solitary hemangioma of the humerus with spontaneous fracture. There was diffuse bleeding at the time of the biopsy. Later the brachial artery was clamped, the tumor resected and replaced with a graft from the bank. Satisfactory healing with good function. (Courtesy of Dr. H. C. Schumm.)

FIG. 303. Multiple Hemangioma

A. B., male, age 5, 5/13/54. Pathologic fracture of the right humerus through a hemangioma. There were multiple lesions and had been innumerable fractures. They healed readily, this one with a hanging cast.

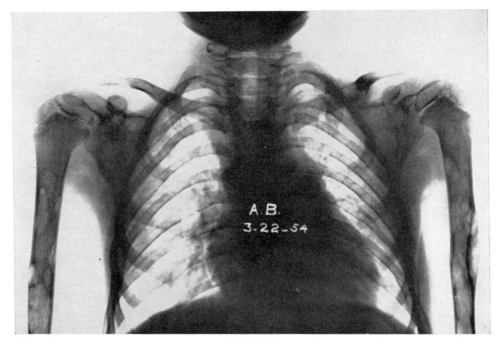

FIG. 304. Multiple Hemangioma

A. and B. A roentgenogram of the case in Figure 303 showing the multiplicity of lesions including ribs, clavicle, scapulae, as well as humerii.

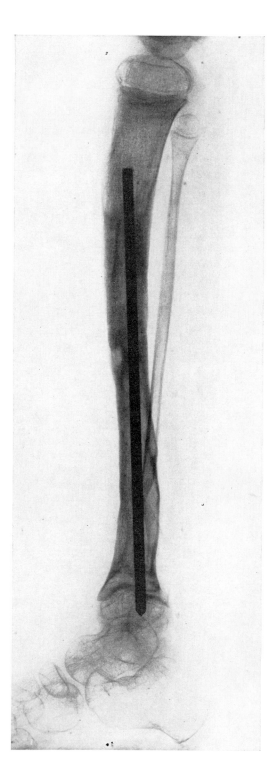

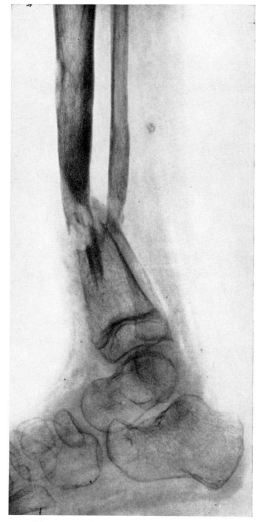

FIG. 305. Congenital Pseudarthrosis

J. B., male, age 7, 10/6/53. Congenital fracture of the tibia following an unsuccessful attempt at bone graft. The deformity was characteristic. [Courtesy of Dr. Harold Sofield (138).]

FIG. 306. Healed Congenital Pseudarthrosis

J. B., 7/2/54. The same leg as in Figure 305 after resection of the pseudarthrosis and rearrangement of the metaphysis to bring healthy bone to the lower third. The defect was filled with bank bone. Almost complete healing. Alignment was maintained by an intramedullary rod. This method offers more hope of permanent cure than some of those previously tried. [Courtesy of Dr. Harold Sofield (138).]

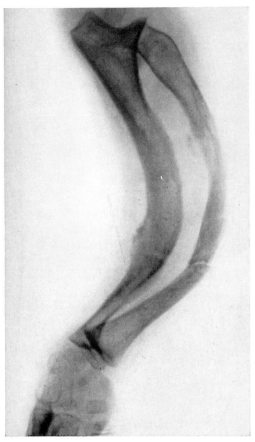

Fig. 307. Osteogenesis Imperfecta
J. N., male, age 8, 11/16/33. Fracture through
the left forearm of a case of osteogenesis imperfecta.
The deformities had increased in severity until the
child died.

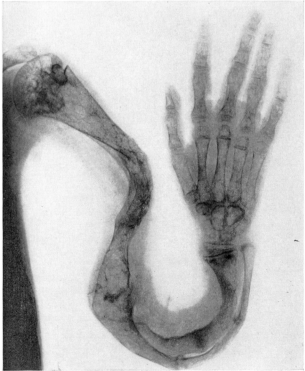

Fig. 308. Osteogenesis Imperfecta
E. K., female, age 8, 5/25/51.
Osteogenesis imperfecta of the severe
type with multiple fractures, extreme
deformity and marked diffuse bone
atrophy. [Courtesy of Dr. Harold
Sofield (138).]

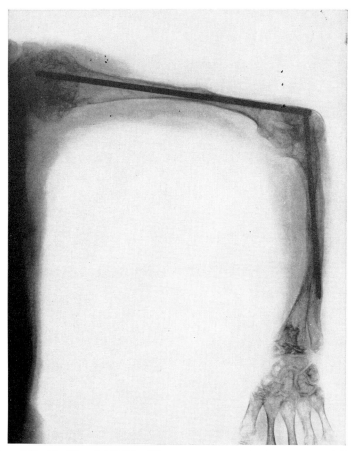

Fig. 309. E. K., 8/26/53. The same arm as in Figure 308 following resection of the shaft and "rodding". The diaphysis was cut into segments, many of them rotated 180° and the bone straightened out. Healing was nearly complete. [Courtesy of Dr. Harold Sofield (138).]

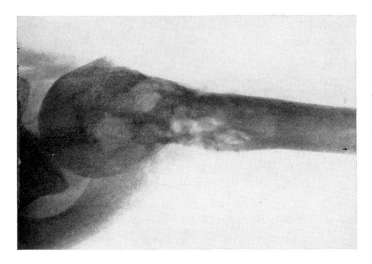

FIG. 310. Eosinophilic Granuloma
M. S., female, age 14, 2/21/49.
Eosinophilic granuloma with a pathologic fracture of the proximal third of
the left humerus. The patient had
had lesions of the left femur, left
ilium, and second lumbar vertebra.
The left humerus was the only bone
to fracture.

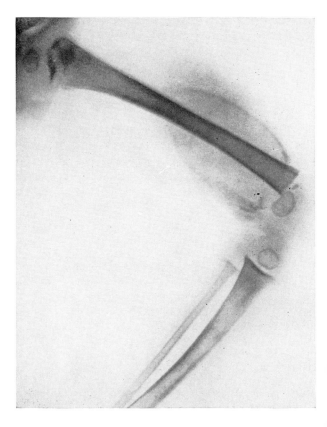

FIG. 311. Infantile Scurvy
S. N., 8/21/28. Healing scurvy in
an infant. Pathologic fracture of the
distal metaphysis of the left femur
with displacement of the epiphysis.
The subperiosteal new bone outlined the hematoma, which later
calcified. The shaft realigned itself
with the epiphysis and eventually it
was straight.

References

1. ASHHURST, A. P. C.: An Anatomical and Surgical Study of Fractures of the Lower End of the Humerus. Philadelphia, Lea & Febiger, 1910.
2. TRUESDELL, E. D.: Birth Fractures and Epiphyseal Dislocations. New York, Paul B. Hoeber, Inc., 1917.
3. HOLLAND, C. T.: Radiographical note on injuries to distal epiphyses of radius and ulna. Proc. Roy. Soc. Med. *22:* 695, 1929.
4. BLOUNT, W. P.: Proximal osteotomies of the femur. Am. Acad. Orthop. Surg. Instructional Course Lectures *9:* 1, 1952. Ann Arbor, J. W. Edwards, Inc., 1952.
5. ODELL, R. T., AND LEYDIG, S. M.: The conservative treatment of fractures in children. Surg., Gynec. & Obst. *92:* 69, 1951.
6. WILSON, P. D.: Capsulectomy for the relief of flexion contractures of the elbow following fracture. J. Bone & Joint Surg. *26:* 71, 1944.
7. BILLINGTON, R. W.: A new (plaster yoke) dressing for fracture of the clavicle. South. Med. J. *24:* 667, 1931.
8. SNEDECOR, S. T., AND WILSON, H. B.: Some obstetrical injuries to the long bones. J. Bone & Joint Surg. *31A:* 378, 1949.
9. MICHEL, L.: Obstetrical dislocation of the upper humeral epiphysis (Le décollement obstétrical de l'épiphyse supérieure de l'humérus). Rev. d' orthop. *24:* 201, 1937. Abstr. Surg., Gynec. & Obst. *65:* 243, 1937.
10. AITKEN, A. P.: End results of fractures of the proximal humeral epiphysis. J. Bone & Joint Surg. *18:* 1036, 1936.
11. CODMAN, E. A.: The Shoulder, p. 41. Boston, T. Todd Co., 1934.
12. BOURDILLON, J. F.: Fracture-separation of the proximal epiphysis of the humerus. J. Bone & Joint Surg. *32B:* 35, 1950.
13. AUSTIN, L. J.: Fractures of the morphological neck of the humerus in children. Canad. Med. Assn. J. *40:* 546, 1939.
14. CAVE, E. F.: Personal communication.
15. BERGENFELDT, E.: Traumatic epiphyseal separation of the long bones of the extremities (Beiträge zur Kenntnis der traumatischen Epiphysenlösungen an den langen Röhrenknochen der Extremitäten: eine klinische-röntgenologische Studie). Acta Chir. Scandinav. (supp. 28) *73:* 149, 1933.
16. WATSON-JONES, R.: Fractures and Joint Injuries, 3rd ed., vol. 2, p. 485. Baltimore, The Williams & Wilkins Co., 1943.
17. ATTENBOROUGH, C. G.: Remodelling of the humerus after supracondylar fractures in childhood. J. Bone & Joint Surg. *35B:* 386, 1953.
18. DUNLOP, J.: Transcondylar fractures of the humerus in childhood J. Bone & Joint Surg. *21:* 59, 1939.
19. ALLEN, P. D., AND GRAMSE, A. E.: Transcondylar fractures of the humerus treated by Dunlop traction: report of 21 cases from Children's Surgical Service, Bellevue Hospital, New York City. Am. J. Surg. *67:* 217, 1945.
20. JONES, R.: On injuries to the elbow-joint. Clin. J. *25:* 17, 1904.
21. CARLI, C.: Wire traction for supra-

condylar fracture of the elbow in children (Trazione col filo nelle fratture sovracondiloidee di gomito del bambino). Chir. d. org. d. movimento *18:* 311, 1933.

22. BLOUNT, W. P.: Volkmann's ischemic contracture. Surg., Gynec. & Obst. *90:* 244, 1950.

23. HARMAN, J. W.: The significance of local vascular phenomena in the production of ischemic necrosis in skeletal muscles. Am. J. Path. *24:* 625, 1948.

24. ALLISON, N.: Fractures about the elbow. J. A. M. A. *89:* 1568, 1927.

25. SEVER, J. W., AND GALLUPE, H. Q.: Fracture of the elbow. J. A. M. A. *98:* 1737, 1932.

26. CHUTRO, P.: Fracturas de la Extremidad Inferior del Humero en los Ninos. Tesis. Buenos Aires, J. Peuser, 1904.

27. DUNN, N.: Supracondylar fracture of the elbow. Brit. Med. J. *2:* 663, 1936.

28. DAVIDSON, A. J., AND HORWITZ, M. T.: Late or tardy ulnar-nerve paralysis. J. Bone & Joint Surg. *17:* 844, 1935.

29. FAIRBANK, H. A. T., AND BUXTON, St. J. D.: Displacement of the internal epicondyle into the elbow-joint. Lancet *2:* 218, 1934.

30. PATRICK, J.: Fracture of the medial epicondyle with displacement into the elbow joint. J. Bone & Joint Surg. *28:* 143, 1946.

31. POTTER, C. M. C.: Fracture-dislocation of the trochlea. J. Bone & Joint Surg. *36B:* 250, 1954.

32. LEWIS, R. W., AND THIBODEAU, A. A.: Deformity of the wrist following resection of the radial head. Surg., Gynec. & Obst. *64:* 1079, 1937.

33. AITKEN, A. P.: In discussion on BEEKMAN, F., AND SULLIVAN, J. E.: Some observations of fractures of long bones in children. Am. J. Surg. *51:* 736, 1941.

34. KEY, J. A.: Treatment of fractures of the head and neck of the radius. J. A. M. A. *96:* 101, 1931.

35. BLOUNT, W. P.: Unusual fractures in children. Am. Acad. Orthop. Surg. Instructional Course Lectures *11:* 57, 1954. Ann Arbor, J. W. Edwards, Inc., 1954.

36. SCHULZ, I.: Fractures of the elbow in children. Wisc. Med. J. *36:* 913, 1937.

37. ZEITLIN, A.: The traumatic origin of accessory bones at the elbow. J. Bone & Joint Surg. *17:* 933, 1935.

38. BOYD, H. B.: Surgical exposure of the ulna and proximal third of the radius through one incision. Surg., Gynec. & Obst. *71:* 86, 1940.

39. EVANS, E. M.: Pronation injuries of forearm with special reference to anterior Monteggia fracture. J. Bone & Joint Surg. *31B:* 578, 1949.

40. BOYD, H. B.: Fractures about the elbow in children. Surg., Gynec. & Obst. *89:* 775, 1949.

41. MAGILL, H. K., AND AITKEN, A. P.: Pulled elbow. Surg., Gynec. & Obst. *98:* 753, 1954.

42. HUTCHINSON, J., JR.: On certain obscure sprains of the elbow occurring in young children. Ann. Surg. *2:* 91, 1885.

43. BOURGUET: So-called incomplete luxation of the proximal end of the radius (Mémoire sur les luxations dites incomplètes de l'extrémité supérieure du radius). Rev. med.-chir. *15:* 287, 1854.

44. VAN ARSDALE, W. W.: On subluxation of the head of the radius in children with a resume of one hundred consecutive cases. Ann. Surg. *9:* 401, 1889.

45. BLOUNT, W. P., SCHULZ, I., AND

CASSIDY, R. H.: Fractures of the elbow in children. J. A. M. A. *146:* 699, 1951.

46. GREEN, J. T., AND GAY, F. H.: Traumatic subluxation of the radial head in young children. J. Bone & Joint Surg. *36A:* 655, 1954.

47. BÖHLER, L.: Treatment of complicated fractures of the forearm (Behandlung schwerer Vorderarmbrüche). Arch. f. klin. Chir. *162:* 713, 1930.

48. LEUVEUF, J., AND GODARD, H.: Bone pegs in fractures of the forearm in children (L'enchevillement osseux dans les fractures de l'avant bras chez l'enfant). J. de Chir. *48:* 792, 1936.

49. BOSWORTH, B. M.: Fractures of both bones of the forearm in children. Surg., Gynec. & Obst. *72:* 667, 1941.

50. WATSON-JONES, R.: Fractures and Joint Injuries, 3rd ed., vol. 2, p. 514. Baltimore, The Williams & Wilkins Co., 1943.

51. GIBERSON, R. G., AND IVINS, J. C.: Fractures of the distal part of the forearm in children: correction of deformity by growth. Minn. Med. *35:* 744, 1952.

52. BLOUNT, W. P., SCHAEFER, A. A., AND JOHNSON, J. H.: Fractures of the forearm in children. J. A. M. A. *120:* 111, 1942.

53. CHARNLEY, J.: The Closed Treatment of Common Fractures, p. 3. Baltimore, The Williams & Wilkins Co., 1950.

54. KEY, J. A., AND CONWELL, H. E.: The Management of Fractures, Dislocations and Sprains, 4th ed., p. 796. St. Louis, C. V. Mosby Co., 1946.

55. SCHULZ, I.: Wringer injury. Surg. *20:* 301, 1946.

56. HAUSMANN, P. F. AND EVERETT, H. H.: Wringer injury. Surg. *28:* 71, 1950.

57. HARDIN, C. A., AND ROBINSON, D. W.: Coverage problems in the treatment of wringer injuries. J. Bone & Joint Surg. *36A:* 292, 1954.

58. MOBERG, E.: Use of traction treatment for fractures of phalanges and metacarpals. Acta chir. scandinav. *99:* 341, 1950.

59. BUNNELL, S.: Surgery of the Hand, 2nd ed. Philadelphia, J. B. Lippincott Co., 1948.

60. FRACKELTON, W. H.: Salvaging the Injured Hand. Milwaukee, Newberry Publ., Inc., in press.

61. *American Society for Surgery of the Hand:* The Care of Hand Injuries. Bulletins, Am. Soc. Surg. Hand, 1949.

62. FLYNN, J. E.: Problems with trauma to the hand. J. Bone & Joint Surg. *35A:* 132, 1953.

63. MASON, M. L.: Primary and secondary tendon suture: discussion of significance of technique in tendon surgery. Surg., Gynec. & Obst. *70:* 392, 1940.

64. CRIKELAIR, G. F., CROWLEY, R. T., AND MILLER, H.: Management of severe trauma to distal digital extremities. Am. J. Surg. *85:* 322, 1953.

65. MALGAIGNE, J. F.: A Treatise on Fractures. Translated from the French by J. H. Packard. Philadelphia, J. B. Lippincott Co., 1859.

66. DESTOT, E.: Pronation and supination of the forearm in traumatic lesions (Pronation et supination de l'avant-bras dans les lesions traumatiques). Presse Med. *21:* 41, 1913.

67. LEVANDER, G.: Treatment of fractures of the shaft of the femur (Ueber die Behandlung von Brüchen des Oberschenkelschaftes). Acta chir. Scandinav. (supp. 12) *65:* 5, 1929.

68. FRIEDRICH, P. L.: The aseptic prepara-

tion of fresh wounds (Die aseptische Versorgung frischer Wunden). Arch. f. klin. Chir. *57:* 288, 1898.

69. BRYANT, T.: The Practice of Surgery, vol. 2, p. 405. London, J. & A. Churchill, 1876.

70. CONWELL, H. E.: Acute fractures of the shaft of the femur in children. J. Bone & Joint Surg. *11:* 593, 1929.

71. RUSSELL, R. H.: Fractures of the femur: a clinical study. Brit. J. Surg *11:* 491, 1924.

72. THOMSON, S. A., AND MAHONEY, L. J.: Volkmann's ischemic contracture: relationship to fracture of the femur. J. Bone & Joint Surg. *33B:* 336, 1951.

73. ASHHURST, A. P. C., AND NEWELL W. A.: Conservative treatment of fractures of the femur. Ann. Surg. *48:* 749, 1908.

74. BLOUNT, W. P.: Blade-plate internal fixation for high femoral osteotomies. J. Bone & Joint Surg. *25:* 319, 1943.

75. MAGNUSON, P. B.: Fractures, 3rd ed., p. 268. Philadelphia, J. B. Lippincott Co., 1939.

76. EHALT, W.: Traction and bed rest for fractures of the femur and tibia in children (Extension und Lagerung bie kindlichen Unterschenkel- und Oberschenkelbrüchen). Chirurg. *21:* 386, 1950.

77. DAVID, V. C.: Shortening and compensatory overgrowth following fractures of the femur in children. Arch. Surg. *9:* 438, 1924.

78. BISGARD, J. D., AND MARTENSON, L.: Fractures in children. Surg., Gynec. & Obst. *65:* 464, 1937.

79. AITKEN, A. P.: Overgrowth of the femoral shaft following fracture in children. Am. J. Surg. *49:* 147, 1940.

80. PHEMISTER, D. B.: Operative arrest of longitudinal growth of bones in the treatment of deformities. J. Bone & Joint Surg. *15:* 1, 1933.

81. BLOUNT, W. P., AND CLARKE, G. R.: Control of bone growth by epiphyseal stapling. J. Bone & Joint Surg *31A:* 464, 1949.

82. HELFERICH, H.: Production of increased new bone formation (Ueber kunstliche Vermehrung der Knochenneubildung). Arch. f. klin. Chir. *36:* 873, 1887.

83. FERGUSON, A. B.: Surgical stimulation of bone growth by a new procedure. J. A. M. A. *100:* 26, 1933.

84. PEASE, C. N.: Local stimulation of growth of long bones. J. Bone & Joint Surge. *34A:* 1, 1952.

85. BLOUNT, W. P., AND ZEIER, F.: Control of bone length. J. A. M. A. *148:* 451, 1952.

86. COLE, W. H.: Compensatory lengthening of the femur in children after fracture. Ann. Surg. *82:* 609, 1925.

87. BLOUNT, W. P., SCHAEFER, A. A., AND FOX, G. W.: Fractures of the femur in children. South. Med. J. *37:* 481, 1944.

88. WILSON, J. C.: Fractures of the neck of the femur in childhood. J. Bone & Joint Surg. *22:* 531, 1940.

89. CARRELL, B., AND CARRELL, W. B.: Fractures of the neck of the femur in children with particular reference to aseptic necrosis. J. Bone & Joint Surg. *23:* 225, 1941.

90. ALLENDE, G., AND LEZAMA, L. G.: Fracture of neck of the femur in children. J. Bone & Joint Surg. *33A:* 387, 1951.

91. INGRAM, A. J., AND BACHYNSKI, B.: Fractures of the hip in children. J. Bone & Joint Surg. *35A:* 867, 1953.

92. GREEN, W. T.: Slipping of upper femoral epiphysis; diagnostic and thera-

peutic considerations. Arch. Surg. *50:* 19, 1945.

93. JOPLIN, R. J.: Slipped capital femoral epiphysis. Am. Acad. Orthop. Surg. Instructional Course Lectures *7:* 210, 1950. Ann Arbor, J. W. Edwards, Inc., 1950.

94. BLOUNT, W. P.: The anvil-retractor. J. Bone & Joint Surg. *25:* 208, 1943.

95. LAMBERT, C. N.: Personal communication.

96. OSGOOD, R. B.: Lesions of the tibial tubercle occurring during adolescence. Boston Med. & Surg. J. *148:* 114, 1903.

97. CHOYCE, C. C.: Traumatic dislocation of the hip in childhood and relation of trauma to pseudocoxalgia. Brit. J. Surg. *12:* 52, 1924.

98. PLATT, H.: Traumatic dislocation of the hip-joint in a child. Lancet *1:* 80, 1916.

99. CLARKE, H. O.: Traumatic dislocation of the hip-joint in a child. Brit. J. Surg. *16:* 690, 1929.

100. ELMSLIE, R. C.: Pseudocoxalgia following traumatic dislocation of the hip in a boy aged four years. J. Orthop. Surg. *1:* 109, 1919.

101. VAN EDEN, P. H.: Results in the treatment of fractures of the shaft of the femur (Behandlungserfolge der Oberschenkelschaftbruche). Acta chir. scandinav. *67:* 320, 1930.

102. LEAVITT, P. H.: Traumatic separation of the lower-femoral epiphysis. New England J. Med. *245:* 565, 1951.

103. LEVINTHAL, D. H.: Old traumatic displacement of the distal femoral epiphysis. J. Bone & Joint Surg. *18:* 199, 1936.

104. KURLANDER, J. J.: Slipping of the lower femoral epiphysis. J. A. M. A. *96:* 513, 1931.

105. GREEN, W. T., AND ANDERSON, M.: Experiences with epiphyseal arrest in correcting discrepancies in length of the lower extremities in infantile paralysis: a method of predicting the effect. J. Bone & Joint Surg. *29:* 659, 1947.

106. CLARKE, H. O.: Fractures of the tibia involving the knee-joint: fracture of the tibial tubercle. Roy. Soc. Med. Proc. *28:* 1043, 1935.

107. BLOUNT, W. P.: Tibia vara: osteochondrosis deformans tibiae. J. Bone & Joint Surg. *19:* 1, 1937.

108. BOEHM, M.: The Human Leg (Das menschliche Bein). Stuttgart, Enke, 1935.

109. BOEHM, M.: The development of juvenile pes valgus. J. Bone & Joint Surg. *12:* 333, 1930.

110. NACHLAS, I. W.: Medial torsion of the leg. Arch. Surg. *28:* 909, 1934.

111. HOLT, J. F., LATOURETTE, H. B., AND WATSON, E. H.: Physiological bowing of the legs in young children. J. A. M. A. *154:* 390, 1954.

112. BREWER, B. J.: Flake fracture of the talus. Presented at the Orthopedic Section, A. M. A., June 3, 1953.

113. CARRUTHERS, F. W., AND LOGUE, R. M.: Treatment of fractures of the pelvis and their complications. Am. Acad. Orthop. Surg. Instructional Course Lectures *10:* 50, 1953. Ann. Arbor. J. W. Edwards, Inc., 1953.

114. MILCH, H.: Ischial apophysiolysis: a new syndrome. Clin. Orthop. *2:* 184, 1953.

115. McLAUGHLIN, H. L.: Personal communication.

116. ASPLUND, G.: A few cases of ischiopubic osteochondritis. Acta chir. scandinav *67:* 1, 1930.

117. ROGERS, W. A.: Treatment of fracture-dislocation of the cervical spine. J. Bone & Joint Surg. *24:* 245, 1942.

118. DAVIS, A. G.: Injuries of the spinal

column. Am. Acad. Orthop. Surg., Instructional Course Lectures *6:* 73, 1949. Ann Arbor, J. W. Edwards, Inc., 1949.

119. BERKHEISER, E. J., AND SEIDLER, F.: Nontraumatic dislocations of the atlanto-axial joint. J. A. M. A. *96:* 517, 1931.

120 WILSON, M. J., MICHELE, A. A., AND JACOBSON, E. W.: Spontaneous dislocation of the atlanto-axial articulation including a report of a case with quadriplegia. J. Bone & Joint Surg. *22:* 698, 1940.

121. HUETER, C.: Anatomic studies of the joints of the extremities of newborns and adults (Anatomische Studien an den Extremitätengelenken Neugeborener und Erwachsener). Virchow's Arch. f. pathol. Anat. *25:* 572, 1862.

122. VOLKMANN, R.: Diseases of the Locomotor System (Die Krankheiten der Bewegungsorgane). In PITHA AND BILLROTH: Handbuch der allgemeinen und speciellen Chirurgie, Bd. 2, Abt. A, S. 694. Stuttgart, Enke, 1869.

123. SARNAT, B. G., AND GREELEY, P. W.: Effect of injury upon growth and some comments on surgical treatment. Plast. & Reconstruct. Surg. *11:* 39, 1953.

124. SMITH, F.: Plastic and Reconstructive Surgery. Philadelphia, W. B. Saunders Co., 1950.

125. GEORGIADE, N. G., MASTERS, F. W., METZGER, J. T., AND PICKRELL, K. L.: Fractures of the mandible and maxilla in children. J. Pediat. *42:* 440, 1953.

126. CAMPBELL, W. C.: Operative Orthopedics, 2nd ed., vol. 2, p. 1593. St. Louis, C. V. Mosby Co., 1949.

127. FREIBERG, A.: Infraction of the metatarsal head. Surg., Gynec. & Obst. *19:* 191, 1914.

128. CALVÉ, J.: A localized affection of the spine suggesting osteochondritis of the vertebral body with the clinical aspects of Pott's disease. J. Bone & Joint Surg. *7:* 41, 1925.

129. BANCROFT, F. W., AND PILCHER, C.: Surgical Treatment of the Nervous System, fig. 21, p. 44; fig. 22, p. 45; fig. 29, p. 60. Philadelphia, J. B. Lippincott Co., 1946.

130. CLEVELAND, D. A.: Anatomic and physiologic aids in neurologic diagnosis. Wisc. Med. J. *40:* 1037, 1941.

131. LYONS, C., ALTEMEIER, W. A., HAMPTON, O. P., AND SNYDER, H. E.: Report of the Committee for the Study of Immunization as Prophylaxis for Tetanus and Gas Gangrene. Am. J. Surg. *87:* 482, 1954.

132. GILL, G. G.: Cause of discrepancy in length of the limbs following tuberculosis of the hip in children; arrest of growth from premature central closure of the epiphysial cartilages about the knee. J. Bone & Joint Surg. *26:* 272, 1944.

133. LICHTENSTEIN, L.: Aneurysmal bone cyst: pathological entity commonly mistaken for giant-cell tumor and occasionally for hemangioma and osteogenic sarcoma. Cancer *3:* 279, 1950.

134. THOMPSON, P. C.: Subperiosteal giant-cell tumor. J. Bone & Joint Surg. *36A:* 281, 1954.

135. BOYD. H. B., AND FOX. K. W.: Congenital pseudarthrosis. J. Bone & Joint Surg. *30A:* 274, 1948.

136. HELFET, A. J.: New conception of parathyroid function and its clinical application: preliminary report on results of treatment of generalized fibrocystic and allied bone diseases

and of rheumatoid arthritis by aluminum acetate. Brit. J. Surg. *27:* 651, 1940.

137. KEY, J. A.: Brittle bones and blue sclera: hereditary hypoplasia of the mesenchyme. Arch Surg. *13:* 523, 1926.

138. SOFIELD, H. A.: Personal communication.

139. CAFFEY, J.: Pediatric X-ray Diagnosis, 2nd ed., p. 739. Chicago, Year Book Publishers, 1950.

140. SCHEUERMANN, H. W.: Kyphosis dor-

salis juvenilie. Ztschr. f. orthop. Chir. *41:* 305, 1921. Abstr. Acta chir. scandinav. *54:* 29, 1922.

141. HATCHER, C. H.: Pathogenesis of localized fibrous lesions in the metaphyses of long bones. Ann. Surg. *122:* 1016, 1945.

142. BLOUNT, W. P.: Fractures in children. Am. Acad. Orthop. Surg. Instructional Course Lectures *7:* 194, 1950.; Ann Arbor, J. W. Edwards Inc., 1950.

143. BLOUNT. W. P.: Fractures in children. Clin. Med. 365, 1952.

Index

Numbers set in roman type refer to text material; numbers set in *italic* type refer to pages on which illustrations appear.